# Laboratory Manual

to accompany

# Rehabilitation Techniques for Sports Medicine and Athletic Training

*Fourth Edition*

**William E. Prentice, Ph.D., P.T., A.T.C.**
*The University of North Carolina at Chapel Hill*

*Prepared by*
**Thomas W. Kaminski, Ph.D., A.T.C./R**
*University of Delaware*

Boston   Burr Ridge, IL   Dubuque, IA   Madison, WI   New York
San Francisco   St. Louis   Bangkok   Bogotá   Caracas   Kuala Lumpur
Lisbon   London   Madrid   Mexico City   Milan   Montreal   New Delhi
Santiago   Seoul   Singapore   Sydney   Taipei   Toronto

## The **McGraw·Hill** Companies

Laboratory Manual to accompany
Rehabilitation Techniques for Sports Medicine and Athletic Training, Fourth Edition
William E. Prentice

Published by McGraw-Hill Higher Education, an imprint of The McGraw-Hill Companies, Inc., 1221 Avenue of the Americas, New York, NY 10020. Copyright © The McGraw-Hill Companies, Inc., 2004. All rights reserved.

This book is printed on acid-free paper.

2 3 4 5 6 7 8 9 0 QPD QPD 0 6 5 4

ISBN 0-07-284286-5

www.mhhe.com

# Preface

Several years ago, after the release of his 3rd edition textbook *Rehabilitation Techniques in Sports Medicine*, I approached Dr. Prentice with my idea for a Laboratory Manual to accompany his book. After much deliberation and conversations with the publishers, the manual became a reality. Interestingly, several of the reviewers for the release of the new 4th edition textbook also suggested having a manual accompany the textbook. With the recent mandates requiring the execution of educational competencies and clinical proficiencies for athletic training students initiated by the Commission on the Accreditation of Allied Health Education Programs (CAAHEP) in conjunction with the Joint Review Committee – Athletic Training (JRC-AT), it seemed only logical to introduce a laboratory manual to accompany Prentice's classic rehabilitation textbook. In fact, most of the chapters in the manual begin with a review of the selected educational competencies and proficiencies in an easy to use manner.

The laboratory manual is arranged to closely mirror the chapters in the textbook. However, each chapter has been devised to provide only a brief review of the principles, with the primary focus being on the students being involved with the "doing." Most courses involving therapeutic rehabilitation are designed with a laboratory ("hands-on") component in mind. This laboratory manual will fit quite nicely into a 15-16 week semester laboratory course and should offer the instructor a logical course sequence. Each chapter has been organized so that the student spends the majority of time involved with practical, "real life" applications. After all, it is the student who needs to become clinically proficient with the rehabilitation skills, techniques, and tests. Additionally, the laboratory exercises rely on the expertise and knowledge of the clinical instructor to safely and effectively demonstrate techniques and critique the students on performance.

Unfortunately, not every possible rehabilitation technique, skill, and/or test is provided for in this manual. However, several of the techniques and skills presented can be modified to fit almost any application. Through the use of case studies in Chapters 16-23 (on "Rehabilitation Techniques for Specific Injuries"), the student will be provided opportunities to put into practice most of the skills, techniques, and tests they have utilized in the preceding chapters in the manual. The intention is that the student's laboratory experience culminates with a level of optimal competency to function in a clinical environment.

# Acknowledgments

I would like to thank Mr. Gary Ward, ATC/R, PT for his assistance in developing the case scenarios found in Chapters 16-23. His clinical expertise and knowledge were invaluable in the creation of the realistic injury scenarios. I appreciate his efforts and dedication to the project.

I would also like to thank the students in the undergraduate Sports Medicine and Athletic Training education program at Southwest Missouri State University for their help in creating the case scenarios and with the critique of the manual.

# Dedication

I would like to dedicate this laboratory manual to my two mentors Mr. Paul Spear (Marietta College) and Dr. David Perrin (UNC @ Greensboro) for giving me the opportunity to grow not only as a person but as an educator and scholar. Words cannot describe the influence you have had on my professional life. Thank you.

I would be remiss if I didn't offer dedication to my students both past and present, who have consistently shaped me as an educator and scholar in ways that are immeasurable. The memories of our time together will be with me for a lifetime. Thanks for constantly challenging me to become a better person.

To my wife Susan and my children Leigh and Adam, thanks for being a constant source of love and support.

# Table of Contents

Preface                                                                iii

Acknowledgments                                                         v

Dedication                                                             vi

Lab 1     The Evaluation Process in Rehabilitation                      1

Lab 2     Developing a Rehabilitation Protocol                          7

Lab 3     Psychological Considerations for Rehabilitation              13

Lab 4     Reestablishing Neuromuscular Control                         19

Lab 5     Restoring Range of Motion and
          Improving Flexibility                                        33

Lab 6     Regaining Muscular Strength,
          Endurance, and Power                                         39

Lab 7     Regaining Postural Stability and Balance                     55

Lab 8     Core Stabilization Training in Rehabilitation                65

Lab 9     Reactive Neuromuscular Training
          (Plyometrics) in Rehabilitation                              72

Lab 10    Open-Versus Closed-Kinetic-Chain
          Exercise in Rehabilitation                                   83

Lab 11    Isokinetics in Rehabilitation                                95

Lab 12    Joint Mobilization and Traction Techniques
In Rehabilitation                                     107

Lab 13    PNF and Other Soft Tissue Mobilization
Techniques in Rehabilitation                          119

Lab 14    Aquatic Therapy in Rehabilitation           133

Lab 15    Functional Progressions and Functional
Testing in Rehabilitation                             144

Lab 16    Rehabilitation of Shoulder Injuries         156

Lab 17    Rehabilitation of Elbow Injuries            163

Lab 18    Rehabilitation of Wrist, Hand, and Finger Injuries    170

Lab 19    Rehabilitation of Groin, Hip, and Thigh Injuries      175

Lab 20    Rehabilitation of Knee Injuries             183

Lab 21    Rehabilitation of Lower-Leg Injuries        191

Lab 22    Rehabilitation of Ankle and Foot Injuries   197

Lab 23    Rehabilitation of Injuries to the Spine     202

# Laboratory Exercise 1

# The Evaluation Process in Rehabilitation

## PURPOSE:

A critical step in the rehabilitation process is performing a thorough clinical assessment in order to define the problem and develop goals. The purpose of this laboratory exercise is to review the concepts associated with the athletic injury evaluation/assessment process. A summary of the SOAP note format of injury documentation will be included. The student will be expected to critically examine the results of their injury assessment so that they can incorporate the information into an effective rehabilitation plan.

## ATHLETIC TRAINING EDUCATIONAL COMPETENCIES:

*Therapeutic Exercise (Cognitive Domain)*

- Describes rehabilitation, functional, and reconditioning progress using follow-up notes, progress notes, SOAP notes, etc.

*Therapeutic Exercise (Psychomotor Domain)*

- Records rehabilitation or reconditioning progress (e.g., follow-up notes, progress notes).

## ATHLETIC TRAINING CLINICAL PROFICIENCIES:

*Assessment and Evaluation (The student will perform record keeping skills while maintaining patient confidentiality)*

- The student will use a standardized record keeping method (e.g., SOAP, HIPS, HOPS).

- The student will select and use injury, rehabilitation, referral, and insurance documentation.

- The student will use progress notes.

*Health Care Administration (The student will demonstrate the ability to perform record keeping skills with sensitivity to patient confidentiality.)*

- The student will use standardized record keeping methods (e.g., SOAP, HIPS, HOPS).

- The student will select and use injury, rehabilitation, referral, and insurance documentation.

- The student will use progress notes.

- The student will organize patient files to allow systematic storage and retrieval.

## REVIEW OF PRINCIPLES:

*Injury Documentation and Assessment Scheme using SOAP Notes*

"SOAP Notes" are a method of providing the student a format that follows an orderly and logical assessment protocol. The SOAP note format was introduced as part of a system of organizing medical records called the problem oriented medical record (POMR).[1]

### S (Subjective)

This portion of the assessment process involves history taking and listening to the athlete/patient subjectively describe the mechanism of injury, previous history, site of pain, etc...

## O (Objective)

The objective clinical findings are the result of the clinician inspecting, palpating and performing any indicated special tests associated with the injury. Accurate documentation of those findings is a critical step in the evaluation process.

## A (Assessment)

This step involves the clinician developing an *impression* as to what they believe is wrong with the athlete/patient, taking in to consideration all of the facts gathered in the "S" and "O" stages of the evaluation process.

## P (Plan)

Relative to rehabilitation, the "plan" step will involve the clinician developing a logical treatment plan to enable a successful outcome of the injury plaguing the athlete/patient. Disposition in all likelihood will involve the implementation of ROM exercises, strengthening routines, muscle endurance programs, proprioception techniques, and general cardiovascular conditioning exercises among other things.

## TEXTBOOK REFERENCE CHAPTER:

Chapter 3

## REFERENCES:

1. Kettenbach, G. 1990. *Writing S.O.A.P. notes.* Philadelphia, PA: F.A. Davis Company.

# LABORATORY EXERCISES:

1. Implement the SOAP note format to summarize your findings from the following three injury scenarios in a concise and effective manner so that a potential rehabilitation plan can be initiated. For each of the steps involved use your imagination and previous experiences to consider the following. (This list is not all inclusive but is meant to "jump start" your thought process.)

- Location of injury
- Complaints and rating of pain
- Previous history
- What is their ultimate goal of rehab?
- Is any swelling, discoloration, deformity present?
- Assess AROM, PROM and RROM
- Perform any special tests associated with the injury situation
- Assess neurovascular function

### *Injury Scenarios*

a) One of your lacrosse athletes complains of acute Achilles tendinitis two days after practice begins.

b) A diver on your swim team has a well documented case of GH joint instability which she has not had surgically repaired and needs treatment advice for a recent subluxation episode.

c) The second basemen on your baseball team reports to the clinic following a week of immobilization for a 4th digit DIP joint dislocation and is anxious to return to competition.

2. For each of the above three scenarios, document your first day treatment/rehabilitation plan with some detail based on your findings.  Give some consideration to the effectiveness of your plan and how will you evaluate the impact of the first day's progress?  Remember to include some recommendations as to:

- Therapeutic modalities
- Medications
- Techniques to improve ROM
- Tools for improving strength
- Functional activities
- Proprioception tasks

# Laboratory Exercise 2

# Developing a Rehabilitation Protocol

## PURPOSE:

Careful thought and consideration for several different variables make developing rehabilitation programs a challenging yet rewarding clinical experience. The purpose of this laboratory exercise is to encourage the student to develop a rehabilitation protocol based on objective and subjective information gleaned during the athletic injury assessment. The student needs to critically think about the assessment findings and apply them in developing a safe, concise, and effective rehabilitation plan.

## ATHLETIC TRAINING EDUCATIONAL COMPETENCIES:

*Therapeutic Exercise (Psychomotor Domain)*

- Demonstrates appropriate methods of evaluating rehabilitation and reconditioning progress and interpreting results.

- Records rehabilitation or reconditioning progress (e.g., follow-up notes, progress notes).

*Psychosocial Intervention and Referral (Psychomotor Domain)*

- Uses motivational techniques with athletes and others involved in physical activity.

- Develops and implements mental imagery techniques for athletes and others involved in physical activity.

*Health Care Administration (Psychomotor Domain)*

- Uses appropriate medical documentation to record injuries and illnesses (client encounters, history, progress notes, discharge summary, physician letters, treatment encounters).

## ATHLETIC TRAINING CLINICAL PROFICIENCIES:

*Assessment and Evaluation (The student will perform record keeping skills while maintaining patient confidentiality.)*

- The student will use a standardized record keeping method (e.g., SOAP, HIPS, HOPS).

- The student will select and use injury, rehabilitation, referral, and insurance documentation.

- The student will use progress notes.

*Psychosocial Intervention and Referral (The student will integrate motivational techniques into the rehabilitation program)*

- The student will simulate the following motivational techniques used during rehabilitation (verbal motivation, visualization, imagery, desensitization).

## REVIEW OF PRINCIPLES:

The design of most rehabilitation plans will give consideration for the following:

**Figure 2.1** Rehabilitation plan flow diagram.

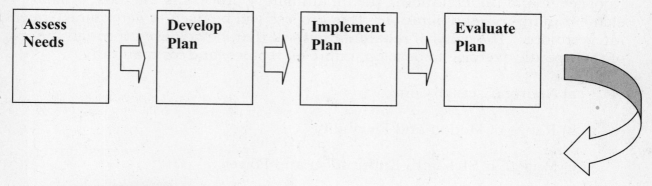

a) **Assess Needs**

- subjective information
- objective data
- list problem areas


b) **Develop Plan**

- establish goals
- select techniques based on available resources
- establish how changes will be documented and monitored
- implement return to play/activity criteria

c) **Implement Plan**

- use procedures and techniques that will fulfill the plan and meet the goals
- incorporate the following psychological components into the plan: verbal motivation, visualization, imagery, desensitization

d) **Evaluate Plan**

- compare original data with current data at frequent intervals
- modify goals according to changes in patient progress and activity level

Knowledge and understanding the inflammatory process is the most crucial element in injury rehabilitation. This process will be used to determine clinical interventions. The goals of rehabilitation will then be achieved through the use of therapeutic exercise to develop, improve, restore, and/or maintain:

a) Neuromuscular Control

b) Range of Motion and Flexibility

c) Muscular Strength, Endurance, and Power

d) Postural Stability and Balance

e) Cardiorespiratory Fitness

## TEXTBOOK REFERENCE CHAPTER:

Chapter 1 & 2

## LABORATORY EXERCISES:

1. Based upon the scheme discussed above, develop a short-term rehabilitation plan based upon the following athletic injury scenarios. (The student should incorporate very specific and logical steps using the previously mentioned principles as a guide.)

   a) A volleyball player with an acute Grade II inversion ankle sprain of the left ankle.

   b) A cross-country runner with a chronic Achilles tendonitis in the right leg.

   c) A softball player with stage I rotator cuff impingement syndrome.

2. Get together with the other students in the lab and determine ways to work with the injured athlete:

a) To improve motivation and exercise compliance

b) To visualize proper technique and performance with certain skills

c) To incorporate imagery techniques into the athlete's rehabilitation plan

# *Laboratory Exercise 3*

# Psychological Considerations for Rehabilitation

## PURPOSE:

There is a belief by some that athletic trainers are 95% psychologist and 5% clinician. As clinicians involved in athletic injury rehabilitation, it is important to give careful consideration to the psychological component of injury healing. The purpose of this laboratory exercise is to have the student develop an awareness of the psychological factors that must be considered to successfully implement a rehabilitation plan. A number of group activities will be utilized for discussion of relevant and contemporary issues as they pertain to athletic injury rehabilitation.

## ATHLETIC TRAINING EDUCATIONAL COMPETENCIES:

*Psychosocial Intervention and Referral (Psychomotor Domain)*

- Communicates with appropriate health care professionals in a confidential manner.

- Uses appropriate community-based resources for psychosocial intervention.

- Uses motivational techniques with athletes and others involved in physical activity.

- Develops and implements stress reduction techniques for athletes and others involved in physical activity.

- Develops and implements mental imagery techniques for athletes and others involved in physical activity.

## ATHLETIC TRAINING CLINICAL PROFICIENCIES:

*Psychosocial Intervention and Referral (The student will integrate motivational techniques into the rehabilitation program.)*

- The student will simulate the following motivational techniques used during rehabilitation: verbal motivation, visualization, imagery, desensitization.

## REVIEW OF PRINCIPLES:

The athletic trainer must be cognizant of both the physical and emotional aspects of return to athletic performance (Figure 3.1).

**Figure 3.1** Physical and psychological factors affecting return to play.

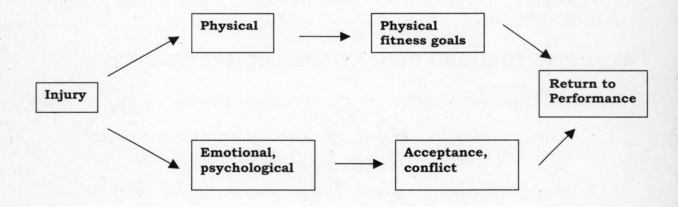

Keep in mind that athletes will react to the injury, rehabilitation, and return to play in very different ways. Some athletes may require interventions for stress reduction along each point of the injury continuum. Some successful intervention strategies can involve the use of buffers, progressive relaxation techniques, and imagery exercises. Additional support may be found with the assistance of an on-campus counseling center, community support groups, or visits with a sport psychologist.

Goal setting is an essential part of the rehabilitation process. Goal setting can aid in the rehabilitation of injured athletes by[1]:

a) Facilitating a faster return to competition

b) Motivating one's effort and persistence

c) Providing a sense of accomplishment

d) Increasing adherence to the rehabilitation program

The following "Guidelines for Goal Setting" were adopted from an article by Wayda and colleagues in 1998 [1]:

1. Goals should be meaningful to both clinician and athlete.

2. Goals must be performance and not outcome oriented.

3. Goals should be individualized for each athlete.

4. Goals must be objective and measurable.

5. Goals must be specific.

6. Goals must include a criterion for success.

7. Goals must be realistic but challenging.

8. Goals must be stated in positive terms.

9. Progressive short-term goals should lead to a long-term goal.

10. Goals should have a target date for completion.

11. Goals should be few and prioritized.

12. Goals should be accompanied by strategies for achievement.

13. Goals must be recorded and monitored.

14. Goals must hold athletes accountable.

15. Goals must be reinforced and supported.

## TEXTBOOK REFERENCE CHAPTER:

Chapter 4

## REFERENCES:

1. Wayda, V.K., F. Armenth-Brothers, and B.A. Boyce. 1998. Goal setting: A key to injury rehabilitation. *Athletic Therapy Today* 3(1): 21-25.

# LABORATORY EXERCISES:

1. Working in groups of 4 or 5 students envision the following "real-life" injury scenarios.

(a) The starting quarterback on your football team suffers a career-ending kidney laceration and is severely depressed upon being released from the hospital.

(b) One of your female field hockey players is quite apprehensive about her upcoming ACLR surgery and lacks confidence in the team orthopaedic surgeon performing the surgery.

e) A softball player who was making excellent progress in her rotator cuff rehabilitation has suffered a recent setback following an infection and is concerned she will not be ready for the start of the Spring season 8 weeks away.

Contemplate and discuss with the other members of your group each of these scenarios and think of:

1) Possible behaviors you might anticipate with each affected athlete;

2) Intervention strategies you as the athletic trainer might employ in these situations; and

3) Potential outcomes that may result of your influence on these situations (both [+] and [-]).

2. Choose a recent athletic injury or surgery you have witnessed. Develop a series of short and long-term goals that are logical and reasonable and can be attained for the individual athlete suffering from that particular malady. Be sure that you provide the specific injury and a historical perspective of the injury.

# *Laboratory Exercise 4*

# Reestablishing Neuromuscular Control

## PURPOSE:

Neuromuscular control is a vital element for success in most athletic endeavors. Consequently, revitalizing the neuromuscular control system becomes an important part of the treatment plan if that system is damaged as a result of injury. The purpose of this laboratory exercise is to review the basic principles associated with reestablishing neuromuscular control and their implications in the rehabilitation process. The student will be expected to execute some basic neuromuscular procedures that can be used in both upper and lower extremity rehabilitation programs.

## ATHLETIC TRAINING EDUCATIONAL COMPETENCIES:

*Therapeutic Exercise (Psychomotor Domain)*

- Demonstrates the appropriate application of contemporary therapeutic exercises including the following:

  • exercises to improve neuromuscular coordination

## ATHLETIC TRAINING CLINICAL PROFICIENCIES:

*Therapeutic Exercise (The student will demonstrate the ability to perform therapeutic exercises.)*

- Exercise to improve neuromuscular control and coordination. The student will demonstrate the ability to instruct the following activities:

### Upper Body:

Rhythmic stabilization
Double- and single-arm balancing
Wobble board or balance apparatus
Weighted-ball rebounding or toss

### Lower Body:

Proprioception board or balance apparatus
Incline board
Single-leg balancing

## REVIEW OF PRINCIPLES:

The following paradigm (Figure 4.1) of the pathophysiology of ligament injury on proprioception and neuromuscular control is based on that presented by Lephart and Henry.[1]

**Figure 4.1** Neuromuscular pathology paradigm.

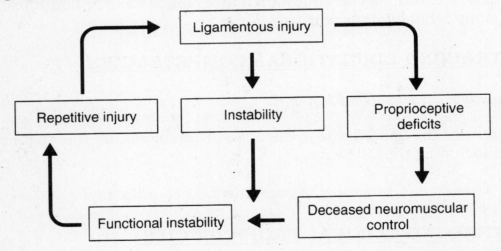

Neuromuscular control activities will work to integrate peripheral sensations relative to joint stimuli and process these signals into a coordinated motor response. Rehabilitation programs should include neuromuscular control activities that will encompass anticipatory (feed-forward) and reflexive (feedback) mechanisms required for normal joint function. The four basic elements for reestablishing neuromuscular control include: joint sensation (position, motion, and force), dynamic stability, preparatory and reactive muscle characteristics, and conscious and unconscious functional motor patterns.[2]

## TEXTBOOK REFERENCE CHAPTER:

Chapter 5

## REFERENCES:

1. Lephart, S.M. and T.J. Henry. 1992. The physiological basis for open and closed chain rehabilitation for the upper extremity. *Journal of Sport Rehabilitation* 5:71-87.

2. Lephart, S.M., C.B. Swanik, F. Fu., and K. Huxel. 2003. Reestablishing neuromuscular control. In *Rehabilitation Techniques in Sports Medicine,* W.E. Prentice, 4th ed. St. Louis: WCB-McGraw Hill.

3. Olmstead, L.C., C.R. Carcia, J. Hertel, and S.J. Shultz. 2002. Efficacy of the Star Excursion Balance Test in detecting reach deficits in subjects with chronic ankle instability. *Journal of Athletic Training* 37(4):495-501.

4. Gribble, P. 2003 The Star Excursion Balance Test: A measurement tool for assessing dynamic balance in research and clinical practice. *Athletic Therapy Today* 8(2):46-47.

5. Tomaszewski, D. 1991. "T-Band Kicks" ankle proprioception program. *Athletic Training, JNATA* 26 (Fall):216-219.

# LABORATORY EXERCISES:

## Neuromuscular Control:

1. <u>Star Excursion Balance Test (SEBT)</u> – The SEBT incorporates a single-leg stance on one leg with maximum reach of the opposite leg (Figure 4.2).[3]

**Figure 4.2** SEBT reach while balancing on the right foot.

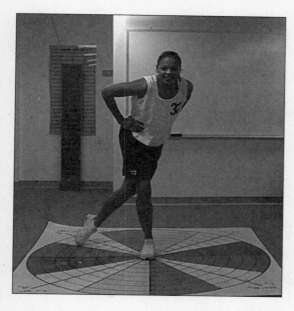

The test is performed with the subject standing at the center of a grid marked on the floor with 8 lines extending 4 feet away from the center at 45° angles. The lines are positioned on the grid and labeled according to the direction of excursion relative to the stance leg (Figure 4.3).[4]

**Figure 4.3** SEBT grid patterns for both right and left leg stances. (Reprinted from Olmstead LC, Carcia CR, Hertel J, Shultz SJ. Efficacy of the Star Excursion Balance Tests in detecting reach deficits in subjects with chronic ankle instability. *J Ath Train.* 2002; 37(4):501-506, Figure 2, The 8 directions of the Star Excursion Balance Tests are based on the stance limb, with permission from the Journal of Athletic Training.)

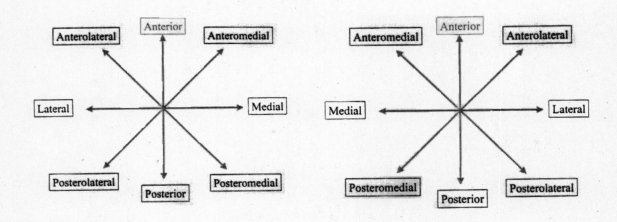

Students should perform the SEBT while working in pairs. One student will score the test while the other student will execute the test. Each student should perform 6 practice trials in each direction to familiarize themselves with the test maneuver. To perform the test each subject will maintain a single-leg stance at the center of the grid with both hands on the hips. They then are instructed with the opposite leg to reach as far as possible along the appropriate vector. The subject is asked to lightly touch the line to ensure that stability is achieved and then return to the upright center position. The distance from the center of the grid to this touch point is measured in centimeters and recorded. A total of 3 reaches/trials along each vector are performed while standing on both the right and left foot. All trials are performed in sequential order working in either a clockwise or counterclockwise direction at the outset. The average of the 3 trials is used in the scoring. Trials are discarded if the subject (1) did not touch the vector line, (2) lifts the stance leg from the center, (3) loses balance, or (4) did not maintain the start and return positions for 1 second. The following scoring template can be used:

**Stance Foot:** _____     **Vector:** _____

**Trial #1 Distance:** _____ (cm)
**Trial #2 Distance:** _____ (cm)
**Trial #3 Distance:** _____ (cm)
**Average Distance:** _____ (cm)

2. "T-Band Kicks" – Rubber elastic bands/tubing can be used to assist with retraining dynamic joint stabilization and to stimulate neuromuscular reflex activity of the lower extremity.[5]  The elastic bands are attached to the distal portion of either limb (involved or uninvolved). The basic patterns involve movements of the hip in flexion/extension (Figure 4.4) and adduction/abduction (Figure 4.5).  As the patient progresses, diagonal patterns can be added.  Additionally, the patient can begin on a stable surface and advance to unstable surfaces (foam, wobble boards, foam rollers, etc...).  The velocity of oscillations can also be changed to increase the difficulty of the activity.  Different sizes of elastic bands and tubing can be used to vary the amount of resistance.

**Figure 4.4**  Hip flexion/extension "T-band" kicks with tubing.

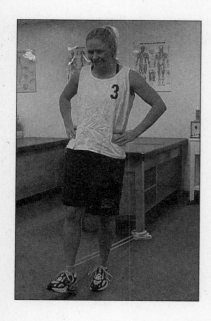

**Figure 4.5** Hip abduction/adduction "T-band" kicks with tubing.

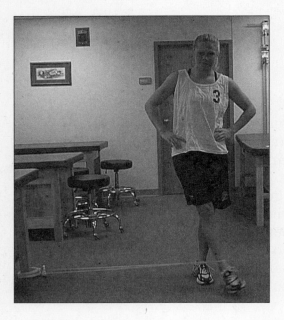

Working with your lab partner, perform a series of "T-Band Kicks" while balancing on one leg at a time. Start with the simple patterns of movement and progress to more advanced routines by influencing the speed of oscillations, adding diagonal motions, and changing surfaces. Perform the routine for 30 seconds, slowly progressing to 1 minute bouts. A metronome can be used to keep pace with a certain beat (i.e. 1 kick every 3 seconds, etc...)

3. <u>Upper Extremity Rhythmic Stabilization</u> – Multidirectional rhythmic stabilization exercises can be performed to facilitate reactive neuromuscular mechanisms in the rehabilitation of upper extremity injuries. Utilizing either manual resistance or elastic bands, the shoulder joint can be loaded in a functional manner to simulate sport activity.

Lab participants should work in pairs to perform the rhythmic stabilization exercises. Begin by using manual resistance to multidirectional movements of the GH joint (Figure 4.6). Each exercise bout should be performed for 30 seconds. Begin with 3-5 repetitions, and gradually build up to performing 10 repetitions. The patient should perform the exercises with maximal effort. Shoulder IROT and EROT patterns may also be used (Figure 4.7). Upon completing the manual exercises, switch to using an elastic band to provide the resistance to movement. Complete these exercises in a similar manner.

**Figure 4.6** Rhythmic stabilization exercise routine for multidirectional movements of the GH joint.

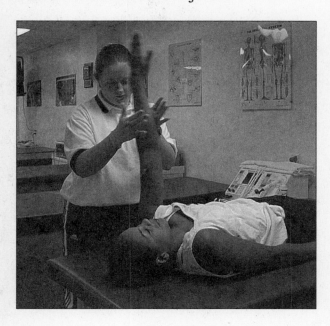

**Figure 4.7** Rhythmic stabilization exercise routine for the GH joint EROT/IROT

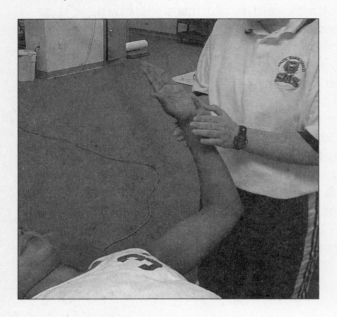

## Proprioception and Kinesthesia:

1. <u>Joint Repositioning</u> – The conscious and unconscious appreciation of joint position best defines proprioception.[2] A variety of joint repositioning activities can be performed to assess this neuromuscular entity. The following assessment tools can be utilized in the laboratory to measure joint position sense:

    a) <u>Goniometric Assessment</u> – The lab can be divided into pairs. One partner will perform the movement while the other partner measures the motion using a goniometer. The test subject will perform a seated knee extension maneuver with the eyes closed. Begin by choosing a target angle between 90° of knee flexion and complete knee extension. Have the subject actively move the knee to the target angle, using the goniometer to monitor (Figure 4.8). Hold the target angle for 5 seconds. The leg is then returned to the start position. The test subject now attempts to reposition the leg to the target angle with the eyes closed. A total of three trials are performed. An error score (degrees) is calculated by subtracting the actual angle from the target angle in each trial. The average absolute error of the three trials is the overall error score. Comparisons can be made between sides or injured vs. uninjured sides. Progression can be made to the assessment of joint position sense in other joints.

**Joint Motion:** _____      **Target Angle:** _____°

Trial #1 Angle ____°      Trial #2 Angle ____°      Trial #3 Angle ____°
Absolute Error = _      Absolute Error = _      Absolute Error = _

**Figure 4.8** Assessing knee extension JPS using a handheld goniometer.

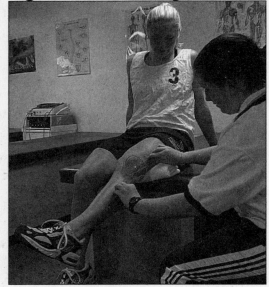

b) <u>Inclinometer Assessment</u> – A simple bubble goniometer (inclinometer) can also be utilized to assess joint repositioning (Figure 4.9). With one partner lying supine on the treatment table, position the arm to assess active shoulder IROT and EROT motions. Blindfold your subject or have them close their eyes. The inclinometer can be secured to the wrist using a Velcro strap. The start position should be a point halfway between full IROT and EROT. Target angles can be selected within the defined range. Trials are then performed in a similar manner as was described above in the goniometric assessment section of the laboratory exercise. Error scores can be compared between motions and sides.

**Arm:** _____    **Joint Motion:** _____    **Target Angle:** _____°

Trial #1 Angle ___°        Trial #2 Angle ___°        Trial #3 Angle ___°
Absolute Error = _         Absolute Error = _         Absolute Error = _

**Figure 4.9** Assessment of GH joint EROT JPS using an inclinometer.

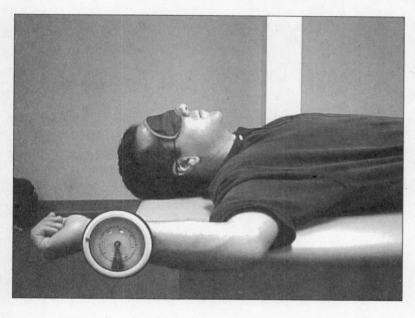

31

c) <u>Isokinetic Dynamometer Assessment</u> – Students having access to isokinetic dynamometers can also assess joint reposition sense using the built-in electrogoniometers equipped on these devices (Figure 4.10). Active and passive joint repositioning can be assessed and measured in degrees of range of motion. The shoulder, knee, and ankle joints are most commonly assessed. The dynamometer's velocity can be set at a point between 0°/sec and 5°/sec. The subject is blindfolded or closes their eyes for the testing. The procedures previously discussed can be utilized once the patient has been positioned on the dynamometer according to the manufacturer's recommendations.

**Figure 4.10** Ankle joint JPS testing using an isokinetic dynamometer.

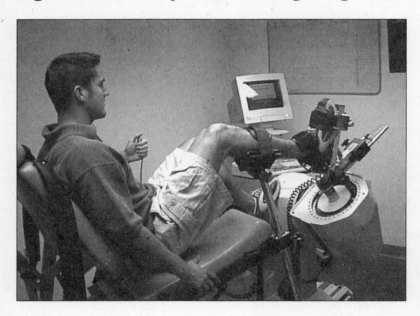

# Laboratory Exercise 5

# Restoring Range of Motion and Improving Flexibility

## PURPOSE:

One of the first steps in the rehabilitation process is the restoration of normal joint range of motion. Without normal ROM, it is very difficult to achieve success with the other rehabilitation goals. The purpose of this laboratory exercise is twofold: to allow the students an opportunity to become proficient at measuring active and passive range of motion and to enable the student an opportunity to work with exercises intended to improve joint ROM and flexibility so that they may be incorporated into a rehabilitation program.

## ATHLETIC TRAINING EDUCATIONAL COMPETENCIES:

*Assessment and Evaluation (Psychomotor Domain)*

- Demonstrates active, passive, and resisted range-of-motion testing of the toes, foot, ankle, knee, hip, shoulder, elbow, wrist, thumb, hand, fingers, and spine.

- Measures active and passive joint range-of-motion with a goniometer.

*Therapeutic Exercise (Psychomotor Domain)*

- Measures the physical effects of injury using contemporary methods (isokinetic devices, goniometers, dynamometers, manual muscle testing, calipers, functional testing) and uses this data as a basis for developing individualized rehabilitation or reconditioning programs.

- Demonstrates the appropriate application of contemporary therapeutic exercises including the following:

  • Passive, active, and active-assisted exercise

## ATHLETIC TRAINING CLINICAL PROFICIENCIES:

*Risk Management and Injury Prevention*

The student will perform fitness tests and record and interpret the data using accepted procedures and equipment.

- The student will demonstrate the ability to perform and evaluate the results of the following tests:

  • Flexibility tests

The student will instruct and demonstrate for the client specific flexibility exercises and activities.

- The student will select range-of-motion exercises and activities for all major muscle groups and their associated joints and instruct a client to perform these exercises. The exercises must include the following body regions and joints:

  • Cervical region
  • Shoulder: joint & girdle
  • Elbow
  • Wrist
  • Hand & fingers
  • Lumbar region
  • Hip & pelvis
  • Knee
  • Leg
  • Ankle
  • Foot & toes

*Assessment and Evaluation*

The student will perform proper clinical evaluation techniques, including range-of-motion testing (active, passive, assisted).

- The student will qualitatively assess active, passive, resistive range-of-motion for the following:

- Temporomandibular joint
- Cervical spine
- Shoulder
- Elbow
- Wrist & hand
- Thumb & fingers
- Hip
- Lumbar spine
- Thoracic spine
- Knee
- Ankle
- Foot & toes

*Therapeutic Exercise*

The student will demonstrate the ability to perform therapeutic exercises.

- Exercise to improve the range-of-motion of the upper extremity, lower extremity, trunk, and cervical spine.

- The student will demonstrate the ability to instruct the following exercises:

- Passive range-of-motion exercises
- Active range-of-motion exercises
- Active-assisted range-of-motion exercises

## REVIEW OF PRINCIPLES:

### Goniometry:

Accurate and reliable range-of-motion (ROM) measurements provide critical assessment and rehabilitation information to the clinician. Typically ROM is assessed in the clinical environment using a device called a goniometer. Goniometers come in many different styles and sizes. Students beginning to use goniometers in clinical practice must become proficient at the technique so that measurements are consistent across clinicians and trials. Students are encouraged to review a variety of informational sources to obtain normative ROM values for the various joints that can be tested using a goniometer. Accuracy in measurement involves proper patient position, goniometer placement, and readings at the end of the arc of motion. Several textbooks are available that are devoted to the measurement of joint motion (goniometry).

### Flexibility Exercises:

Flexibility in joints and muscles has long been a part of physical fitness. Although a direct link to injury prevention has not been well-established, the maintenance of adequate muscle and joint flexibility allows for normal performance and function. Several techniques for enhancing flexibility have been advocated. The different techniques include ballistic stretching, static stretching, and proprioceptive neuromuscular facilitation (PNF) techniques. The focus of this chapter will be on static stretching techniques. Static stretching involves passively stretching the antagonist muscle at an extended range-of-motion and holding it in place for a period of time (15 – 30 seconds). Static stretches can be performed both actively and passively. Passive techniques may require the assistance of a clinician, partner, or stretching device (T-bar, towel, rubber tubing, etc...). Most static stretches are performed with 3-5 repetitions.

## TEXTBOOK REFERENCE CHAPTER:

Chapter 6

# LABORATORY EXERCISES:

1. Students should secure a large, medium, and small-sized goniometer for this laboratory activity.  Working in pairs, students should become proficient at measuring *active* ROM in the various joints listed below.  Students should try to perform these measurements while the patient is positioned in a variety of gravity dependent (standing) and gravity-eliminated (seated or lying) situations.  It is recommended that students have available a reference source of normative active ROM values for the joints to be measured.  For each joint perform a total of three (3) measurement trials.  Be sure to document your findings using the template below as a guide.  The objective of this assignment is to see how accurate you can become on the repeated trials between yourself (intratester reliability) and your partner (intertester reliability).

  a) Shoulder (flexion, extension, abduction, IROT, EROT)

  b) Elbow (flexion)

  c) Forearm (pronation, supination)

  d) Wrist (flexion, extension, abduction, adduction)

  e) Hip (flexion, extension, abduction, adduction, IROT, EROT)

  f) Knee (flexion, extension)

  g) Ankle (plantar flexion, dorsiflexion)

  h) Foot (inversion, eversion)

## *ROM Measurement Template*

Joint _____          Motion _____

Patient Position: _____

Trial #1 _____°          Trial #2 _____°          Trial #3 _____°

Average ROM Measurement = _____

2. Athletic trainers are often called upon to assist athlete's pre or post practice with a variety of single-muscle stretches. Additionally, these static stretches can be incorporated into various rehabilitation programs as a means of maintaining or improving joint ROM. With a partner, work to improve your technique for stretching out the following joints/muscles:

a) Rotator Cuff (IROT & EROT)

b) Triceps

c) Back Extensors

d) Hamstrings

e) Quadriceps

f) Hip Flexors

g) Gastroc-Soleus Complex

h) Hip Adductors

i) Tensor Fascia Latae & IT Band

j) Piriformis

Instruct your partner/patient to hold each stretch for 15-30 seconds. Have the patient perform a total of 3 stretches for each muscle isolated.

Working together as a group, have each of the students share different stretching techniques that may have proven useful in their own clinical experiences. Challenge yourself to think of the muscle(s) that might be influenced by the various stretching techniques demonstrated. Use your imagination and knowledge of anatomy to experiment with different stretching positions and ways to isolate difficult muscle groups.

# Laboratory Exercise 6

# Regaining Muscular Strength, Endurance, and Power

## PURPOSE:

A fundamental component of any rehabilitation program is the establishment of muscular strength and endurance. Adequate muscle strength is a prerequisite for most of the other aspects of rehabilitation and physical fitness. The purpose of this laboratory exercise is to insure that the athletic training student has the necessary clinical skills to safely and effectively implement muscular strength and endurance routines into the rehabilitation plan. Students will be given ample opportunity to improve upon and refine their clinical techniques while working with a variety of strength enhancement tools. The focus of this chapter will be on manual resistance as well as free-weight training techniques. Isokinetic strengthening will be introduced in a later chapter.

## ATHLETIC TRAINING EDUCATIONAL COMPETENCIES:

*Risk Management and Injury Prevention (Psychomotor Domain)*

- Operate contemporary isometric, isotonic, and isokinetic strength testing devices.

- Provides supervision and instruction to an individual in the use of commercial weight training equipment.

*Therapeutic Exercise (Psychomotor Domain)*

- Measures the physical effects of injury using contemporary methods (isokinetic devices, goniometers, dynamometers, manual muscle testing, calipers, functional testing) and to use this data as a basis for developing individualized rehabilitation or reconditioning programs.

- Demonstrates the appropriate application of contemporary therapeutic exercises including the following:

  • Isometric, isotonic, and isokinetic exercise
  • Eccentric versus concentric exercise
  • Elastic, mechanical, and manual resistance exercise

- Demonstrates the proper techniques for the performance of commonly prescribed rehabilitation and reconditioning exercises.

## ATHLETIC TRAINING CLINICAL PROFICIENCIES:

*Risk Management and Injury Prevention*

The student will perform anthropometric measurement techniques and other appropriate examination and screening procedures.

  - The student will assess the following:

  • Limb girth

The student will perform fitness tests and record and interrupt the data using accepted procedures and equipment.

  - The student will demonstrate the ability to perform and evaluate the results of the following tests:

  • Strength (repetition) testing

The student will operate and instruct the use of isometric, isotonic, and isokinetic weight training equipment.

  - The student will demonstrate the ability to establish repetition maximum (RM) tests.

  - The student will perform isometric tests for the following parts of the body:

- Ankle
- Foot/toes
- Knee
- Hip
- Trunk/torso
- Shoulder
- Elbow
- Wrist
- Hand/fingers

The student will perform the following tests:

- Upper body strength test
- Lower body strength test
- Upper body power test
- Lower body power test
- Upper body muscular endurance test
- Lower body muscular endurance test

*Therapeutic Exercise*

The student will demonstrate the ability to perform therapeutic exercises.

- Exercise to improve muscular strength

  - The student will demonstrate the ability to instruct exercises for the following parts of the body using isometric and progressive resistance techniques:

    - Lower extremity
    - Upper extremity
    - Cervical spine
    - Trunk and torso

## REVIEW OF PRINCIPLES:

### Girth Measurements:

Atrophy often accompanies athletic injury. Clinicians can assess atrophy and monitor the effects of strength training interventions with girth measurements. Often, girth measurements are taken prior to the development of the rehabilitation program to provide the clinician with a starting point and the patient with a basis for improvement. The measurements are then repeated at consistent intervals throughout as a way of monitoring progress toward intended goals. Increases and decreases in girth are thought to have a direct relationship with muscle strength.[1] Girth measurements are typically taken using a standard tape measure. The amount of tension placed on the tape measure during girth assessment may affect the measurements, so Gulick™ spring-loaded devices can be attached to one end (Figure 6.1).

**Figure 6.1** Taking thigh girth measurements with a Gulick™ tape measure.

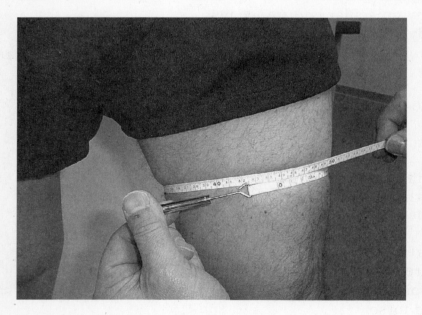

These devices can assist the clinician in applying a known amount of tension with each measurement. In an attempt to insure accurate and reliable measurements the clinician should use the same anatomical landmarks/locations when performing girth measurements. Additionally, some recommend that the muscle should be contracted when taking the measurements.[1]  Girth assessments are commonly performed on the thigh and ankle regions.  In the ankle a figure-8 girth measurement technique is recommended (Figure 6.2).

**Figure 6.2**  The Figure-8 girth measurement technique in the ankle.

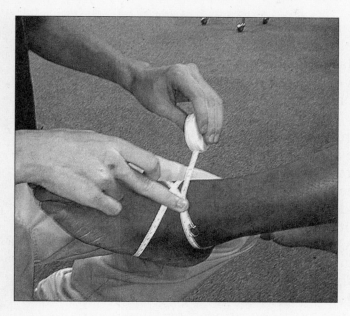

## Muscle Strength Assessment:

The ability for a muscle or muscle group to provide force against some resistance defines muscle strength.  Strength training can be accomplished with isometric, isotonic, and isokinetic training routines.  Three major principles guide most strength training programs.   They include: overload, progressive resistance, and specificity.

Isotonic strength training routines are often introduced into rehabilitation programs to improve strength.  Isotonic muscle movements usually involve accommodations for sets and repetitions.  In order for the clinician to develop an isotonic strength training routine they must first establish the patient's one-repetition maximum (1-RM).  The 1-RM is the maximal amount of weight that a muscle or muscle group can lift one time.  In a clinical setting this may be performed for the quadriceps (knee extension), hamstring (knee flexion), shoulder rotator cuff (IROT and EROT), and ankle plantar flexion muscle groups.  Various systems of strength training are available to the clinician for use in an injury rehabilitation program.  It is suggested that the clinician become comfortable with several techniques and make adjustments to fit the individual patient's needs as the program is initiated. The student is encouraged to review the different strength training systems used in the clinical setting, especially the DeLorme program, Oxford technique, DAPRE program, and Light-to-Heavy system.

Strength training in a clinical setting can be accomplished through the use of several "tools" made available to the clinician. Perhaps the most economical and easiest "tool" to use is your hands. Manual resistance techniques can be adapted to provide resistance to most joint and muscle movements. The same principles that apply to manual muscle testing (MMT) will also work well with manual resistance strength training. Typically, manual resistance exercises are initiated early in the rehabilitation program prior to the patient progressing to advanced resistive loads using free weight equipment, commercial weight machines, or isokinetic dynamometers. Manual resistance techniques can also be used to perform isometric exercises during the strength phase of rehabilitation. Isometric holds should be performed with the patient maintaining the action for 6-10 seconds. These should be repeated 5-10 times. The clinician should also become familiar with the various commercial weight devices available for strength training. These devices can be used to assist strength training at more advanced phases in the rehabilitation process. The same principles and techniques employed with manual and isometric strength training should be incorporated with the routines utilized on these machines.

## Local Muscular Endurance and Power:

Local muscular endurance is the ability of a muscle or muscle group to perform repeated contractions against a light (submaximal) load for an extended period of time.[2] Generally speaking, muscular endurance and muscle strength are linearly related in that as strength improves, so too does endurance. Like strength, muscular endurance is an essential component of the rehabilitation process. There are several local muscular endurance tests that the clinician can utilize to effectively measure endurance, including timed sit-ups, timed push-ups, and maximal repetition chin-ups. Each of these tests provides a unique view on local muscular endurance for either the upper or lower extremity.

Power is the product of the force exerted (strength) on an object and the velocity (speed) of the object in the direction in which the force is exerted.[3] Power is the mathematical product of force and velocity. In sports, some athletic movements are low-speed with high resistive forces, while still others are high-speed with low resistive forces. The clinician needs to have an understanding of the athlete's activity demands and train for power appropriately. The vertical jump is an suitable measure of generalized lower extremity anaerobic power.

## TEXTBOOK REFERENCE CHAPTER:

Chapter 7

## REFERENCES:

1. Harrelson, G.L. 1998. Measurement in rehabilitation. In *Physical Rehabilitation of the Injured Athlete,* J.R. Andrews, G.L. Harrelson, K.E. Wilk. 2nd ed. pp. 55-56. Philadelphia: W.B. Saunders Company.

2. Baumgartner, T. and A. Jackson. 1987. *Measurement and evaluation in Physical Education and Exercise Science.* Dubuque, IA: Brown.

3. Dudley, G.A. and R.T. Harris. 1994. Neuromuscular adaptations to conditioning. In *Essentials of Strength Training and Conditioning,* T.R. Baechle ed. pp. 28-29. Champaign, IL: Human Kinetics.

4. Whitney, S.L., L. Mattocks, J.J. Irrgang, et al. 1995. Reliability of lower extremity girth measurements and right- and left-side difference. *Journal of Sport Rehabilitation* 4:108-115.

5. Esterson, P.S. 1979. Measurement of ankle joint swelling using a Figure of 8. *Journal of Orthopedic and Sports Physical Therapy* 1(1):51-52.

# LABORATORY EXERCISES:

1. The student should become proficient in taking the girth measurements with a variety of cloth, plastic, and metal tape measures. If available, students should also experiment with using a Gulick™ tape measure and work to effectively apply the same tension (4 oz.) with each successive measurement. Working with your partner from class, obtain girth measurements from the following locations:

- Thigh (6 cm and 9 cm above the knee joint line)
- Calf (6 cm and 9 cm below the knee joint line)
- Ankle Figure-8 technique [5]
- Biceps (measured at point of greatest circumference both with arm fully flexed and extended)
- Forearm (measured at the point of greatest circumference between elbow and wrist)

Obtain three (3) measurements from each location on both extremities. Record all measurements in centimeters (cm). In healthy individuals, bilateral circumference comparisons should be within 1.5 cm.[4]

**Girth Measurement Template**:

Location: _____          Side: _____

Measure #1 = _____          Measure #2 = _____

Measure #3 = _____          Average  = _____

How do your measurements compare side to side and between each measurement?

What might the thigh and calf girth measurements look like in someone post-ACLR surgery?

2. Instruct your lab partner on how to perform the following strength rehabilitation exercises. Make considerations for demonstrating to them the correct form, proper position, and precise number of sets and repetitions that they are to perform. Some of these exercises may require the use of cuff weights of various sizes or the use of commercial weight devices (if available).

- Quad sets
- Ham sets
- Calf raises
- Straight leg raises (SLR's)
- Short-arc quads (SAQ's)
- Empty-can shoulder exercises
- Shoulder IROT and EROT exercises
- Hamstring curl and knee extension exercises on a weight machine
- Towel gathering exercises for the foot intrinsics
- Rubber tubing exercises for the following joints (ankle, knee, hip, shoulder, and elbow)
- Leg-press exercises on a commercial weight device.
- Hamstring leans (eccentric hamstring lowering exercises)

3. Manual therapy techniques are quite useful in early stage rehabilitation for a variety of joint injuries. Using your knowledge and skills of manual muscle testing (MMT), perform manual resistance exercises for the following joints:

- Ankle (inversion/eversion, plantar flexion/dorsiflexion)
- Knee (flexion/extension)
- Hip (abduction/adduction, flexion/extension, IROT/EROT)
- Shoulder (abduction/adduction, flexion/extension, IROT/EROT)
- Elbow (flexion/extension)

Work to develop your ability to monitor and change your resistive force. Note the importance of proper positioning and stabilization so that you as the clinician do not become too fatigued during the administration of these rehabilitation activities.

What joint motions required more resistive force? and less?

What muscle(s) or joint motions required greater resistive effort? and less?

4. The student should demonstrate proficiency in administering each of the following muscle strength and endurance tests:

- ## Grip Strength Test with a Hand Dynamometer.

This test measures the static strength of the grip squeezing muscles. Adjust the dynamometer so that it fits comfortably in the hand. The fingers should be allowed to flex in such a way that they grip the handle effectively. The subject should grip with maximum effort, holding the dynamometer out in front of them for 2-3 seconds (Figure 6.3). Two (2) readings (in kg) should be taken on both hands. The maximum readings for each hand are summed together for a total composite score. Students should refer to the table of normative values for comparison (Figure 6.4).

**Figure 6.3**

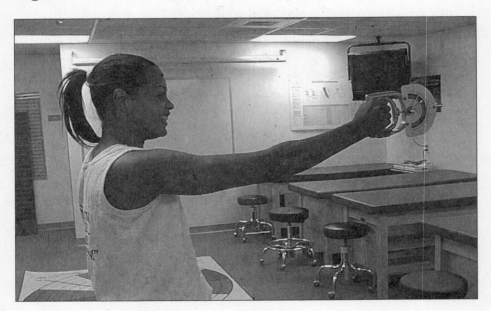

*Right hand*: Trial 1: _____ kg, Trial 2: _____ kg.

*Left hand*: Trial 1: _____ kg, Trial 2: _____ kg.

Your total score is the **sum** of the best trial for each hand.

*Right hand* best trial score = _____ kg

*Left hand* best trial score = _____ kg

Total Score = _____kg

**Figure 6.4** Normative grip strength values for females and males ranging in age from 15-69 years.

### Grip Strength* ( kg)

| Men | | Needs Improvement | Fair | Good | Very Good | Excellent |
|-----|-----|-------------------|------|------|-----------|-----------|
| | 15-19 | Below 84 | 84-94 | 95-102 | 103-112 | Above 112 |
| | 20-29 | Below 97 | 97-105 | 106-112 | 113-123 | Above 123 |
| | 30-39 | Below 97 | 97-104 | 105-112 | 113-122 | Above 122 |
| Age: | 40-49 | Below 94 | 94-101 | 102-109 | 110-118 | Above 118 |
| | 50-59 | Below 87 | 87-95 | 96-101 | 102-109 | Above 109 |
| | 60-69 | Below 79 | 79-85 | 86-92 | 93-101 | Above 101 |

| Women | | Needs Improvement | Fair | Good | Very Good | Excellent |
|-------|-----|-------------------|------|------|-----------|-----------|
| | 15-19 | Below 54 | 54-58 | 59-63 | 64-70 | Above 70 |
| | 20-29 | Below 55 | 55-60 | 61-64 | 65-70 | Above 70 |
| | 30-39 | Below 56 | 56-60 | 61-65 | 66-72 | Above 72 |
| Age: | 40-49 | Below 55 | 55-58 | 59-64 | 65-72 | Above 72 |
| | 50-59 | Below 51 | 51-54 | 55-58 | 59-64 | Above 64 |
| | 60-69 | Below 48 | 48-50 | 51-53 | 54-59 | Above 59 |

*Combined right and left hand grip strength.

SOURCE: *The Canadian Physical Activity, Fitness and Lifestyle Appraisal: CSEP's Plan for Healthy Active Living,* 2nd edition, 1998. Reprinted with permission from the Canadian Society for Exercise Physiology.

- ### 1-RM Test for Strength

Muscular strength in the major muscle groups can be assessed using the 1-RM value. Traditionally, the bench press 1-RM test for strength has been used as a general measure of upper extremity strength. However, in a clinical setting, 1-RM strength values are needed to assess strength in a variety of other muscle groups in the upper and lower extremity. Choose either a biceps curl (elbow flexion) or knee extension (quadriceps) activity and determine your patients 1-RM value. Begin by positioning and stabilizing the patient for the exercise to be performed. Next instruct the patient in the exact maneuver to be executed and to *"breathe in"* as the weight is lowered and *"breathe out"* during the lifting phase of the exercise. Free weights should be used with the clinician close by for intervention if necessary. The weight is adjusted accordingly with each successive repetition. Allow as many trials as needed to achieve the "true" maximum effort. Only one (1) trial is necessary at each weight. Incorporate a 1 – 3 minute rest between trials. Most training schemes will use a percentage of the 1-RM value to determine a starting weight for strength training exercises.

- ### Traditional Pull-Ups (Chin-Ups)

This test is used to assess muscular strength and endurance of the arms and shoulder girdle. The subject begins with the hands facing outward (palms outward) gripping the bar and hanging straight down (Figure 6.5). The body is pulled upward until the chin crosses over the bar. The score is the total number of pull-ups completed until exhaustion. Students should refer to a table of normative values for comparison.

Total pull-up score = _____

**Figure 6.5** Starting position for traditional pull-up.

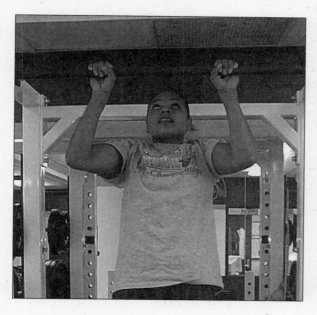

- <u>Vertical Jump for Anaerobic Power</u>

This test can be performed using either a wall scale or commercial vertical jump device. Reach distance while standing on both feet is calculated by measuring from the floor to fingertip. This distance is then subtracted from the jump distance and recorded as the vertical jump. The subject is instructed to perform three (3) trials from a two-footed take-off stance (Figure 6.6).

**Figure 6.6** Subject executing a vertical jump using the Vertec™ (Sports Imports, Columbus, OH) device.

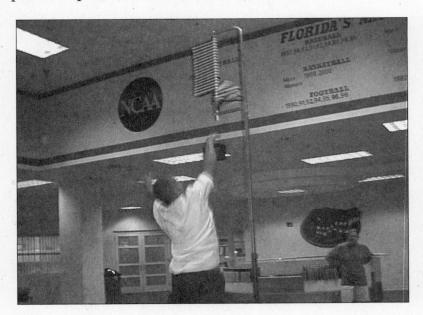

Reach Distance (cm) _____

Trial 1 Jump Height = _____ cm --- VJ #1 = _____ cm

Trial 2 Jump Height = _____ cm --- VJ #2 = _____ cm

Trial 3 Jump Height = _____ cm --- VJ #3 = _____ cm

Average Vertical Jump Height = _____ cm

How does your VJ value compare with others in the class?

What factors will affect VJ performance?

# Laboratory Exercise 7

# Regaining Postural Stability and Balance

## PURPOSE:

Balance is the single most important element dictating movement strategies within the closed kinetic chain.[1]  Most athletic endeavors require the maintenance or acquisition of balance for successful performance and execution.  The purpose of this laboratory exercise is to enable the student an opportunity to work with and effectively initiate a balance assessment and to safely instruct the athlete/patient on balance-training exercises.

## ATHLETIC TRAINING EDUCATIONAL COMPETENCIES:

*Therapeutic Exercise (Psychomotor Domain)*

- Measures the physical effects of injury using contemporary methods (isokinetic devices, goniometers, dynamometers, manual muscle testing, calipers, functional testing) and uses this data as a basis for developing individualized rehabilitation or reconditioning programs.

- Demonstrates the appropriate application of contemporary therapeutic exercises including the following:

- Exercises to improve neuromuscular coordination and proprioception

- Demonstrates the proper techniques for the performance of commonly prescribed rehabilitation and reconditioning exercises.

# ATHLETIC TRAINING CLINICAL PROFICIENCIES:

*Therapeutic Exercise (The student will demonstrate the ability to perform therapeutic exercises.)*

- Exercise to improve neuromuscular control and coordination. The student will demonstrate the ability to instruct the following activities:

### Upper Body:

Rhythmic stabilization
Double- and single-arm balancing
Wobble board or balance apparatus
Weighted-ball rebounding or toss

### Lower Body:

Proprioception board or balance apparatus
Incline board
Single-leg balancing

# REVIEW OF PRINCIPLES:

Balance is the process of maintaining the center of gravity (COG) within the body's base of support.[1] Postural control involves a complex array of feed-forward and feedback mechanisms from both the central and peripheral nervous systems. Balance is considered to be both a static and dynamic process.[1] Effective balance requires input from visual (sight), vestibular (hearing), and somatosensory (body orientation) mechanisms as well as coordinated motions at the hip, knee and ankle.

Balance can be evaluated in a clinical environment via a number of subjective and objective ways. The Romberg test and its many variations are perhaps the most recognized balance assessment tests; however more recently the Balance Error Scoring System (BESS) has proven to be both useful and reliable, especially to those clinicians who cannot afford the expensive balance technology.[2] A wide array of objective balance assessment tools are available, ranging from the less-expensive force plate systems to the more sophisticated systems having both static and dynamic test capabilities.

Because balance depends heavily on coordinated movements in the hip, knee and ankle it is essential that these regions have adequate muscular strength. In addition, appropriate neuromuscular coordination and control are necessary for the maintenance of balance. It is important then for the clinician to keep these two factors is mind when incorporating balance activities into the rehabilitation plan. Balance training activities should involve exercises that:[1]

- Are safe, yet challenging
- Stress multiple planes of motion
- Incorporate multiple sensory systems
- Begin with static, bilateral, and stable surfaces and progress to more dynamic, unilateral, and unstable surfaces
- Proceed to sport specific actions

## TEXTBOOK REFERENCE CHAPTER:

Chapter 8

## REFERENCES:

1. Guskiewicz, K.M. 2003. Regaining balance and postural equilibrium. In *Rehabilitation Techniques in Sports Medicine,* W.E. Prentice, 4th ed. pp. St. Louis: WCB-McGraw Hill.

2. Riemann B.L. K.M. Guskiewicz, E. Shields. 1999. Relationship between clinical and forceplate measures of postural stability. *Journal of Sport Rehabilitation* 8:71-82.

## LABORATORY EXERCISES:

1. The clinical assessment of balance is necessary for the clinician to gain an understanding of the capabilities of the injured patient involved in the rehabilitation program. The student should work to become proficient at administering the following balance tests traditionally used in a clinical setting. Perform several trials with each test to become proficient at scoring and administering the tests appropriately. Compare your scores with those taken by your classmates.

Romberg Test

The simplest of the balance tests, this test is performed with the subject standing on both feet approximately shoulder-width apart (Figure 7.1). The hands are held to the hips (iliac crest). If closing the eyes increases the patient's unsteadiness it is considered a positive (+) test. Most athletes are able to perform this maneuver with relative ease, so several variations to the test have been developed to challenge the postural control systems more effectively.

**Figure 7.1** The Romberg test.

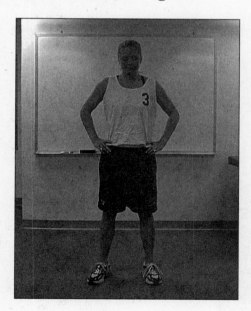

## Unilateral Romberg Test (Modified Romberg, Stork Stand)

This test requires the patient to stand on one foot (injured vs. uninjured) only. The contralateral leg is held tight to the test leg and bent to 45° of knee flexion while the hands are held to the hips (iliac crest) (Figure 7.2). The patient is instructed to hold "steady" in this position for a period of between 20-30 seconds. If the patient loses their balance, they are instructed to make the necessary adjustments and return to the testing position as quickly as possible. The test should be performed with the eyes open and eyes closed. The test can be performed with and without shoes. Error scores are based on any of the following and scored as 1 error point:

- Hands move away from the hips for balance
- Contralateral limb "touches down"
- Contralateral limb moves away from the test leg
- Excessive (> 4") sway occurs
- Open eyes in the eyes closed condition

Small corrections occurring in the ankle, knee, hip, arms, and trunk may occur and are considered normal

**Figure 7.2** Modified Romberg test stance.

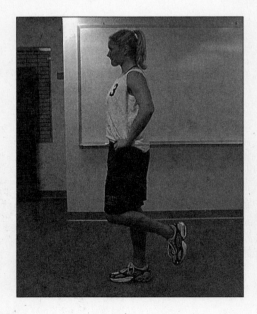

## Sharpened Romberg (Heel-Toe Tandem Stance)

This test requires the patient to stand with one foot in front of the other as if standing on a straight line. The test should be conducted with each foot being in the lead position. The knees and hips should be extended and the patient should attempt to maintain good upright posture while the hands are placed on the hips (iliac crest) (Figure 7.3). The patient is instructed to hold "steady" in this position for a period of between 20-30 seconds. If the patient loses their balance, they are instructed to make the necessary adjustments and return to the testing position as quickly as possible. The test should be performed with the eyes open and closed. The test can be performed with and without shoes. Error scores are based on any of the following and scored as 1 error point:

- Hands move away from the hips for balance
- Contralateral limb "touches down"
- Contralateral limb moves away from the test leg
- Excessive (> 4") sway occurs
- Open eyes in the eyes closed condition

Small corrections occurring in the ankle, knee, hip, arms, and trunk may occur and are considered normal.

**Figure 7.3** The sharpened Romberg stance.

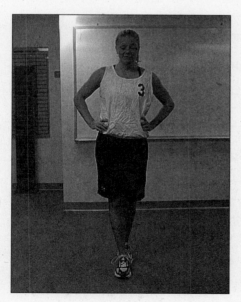

## Balance Error Scoring System (BESS)

Recently the BESS was developed as a cost-effective alternative to computerized balance assessments.[2] The three (3) stance variations of the Romberg test (double, single, tandem) are performed on a firm and foam surface (Figure 7.4). Each test is conducted with the **eyes closed** for 20 seconds each. Two (2) trials are performed with each stance and surface. The BESS is scored as follows:

- Lifting hands off iliac crest
- Opening eyes
- Stepping, stumbling, or falling
- Remaining out of the test position for more than 5 seconds
- Moving hip into more than 30° of flexion or abduction
- Lifting forefoot or heel

The BESS score is calculated by adding one error point for each error or combination of errors occurring during one movement (i.e. lift hands and open eyes = 1 error point). Average error scores from each of the 6 test trials are added together for a total BESS score. Higher scores represent poor balance.

1) **Stance** = Double     **Surface** = Firm
Trial 1 Error Score = _____
Trial 2 Error Score = _____
Average Error Score = _____

2) **Stance** = Double     **Surface** = Foam
Trial 1 Error Score = _____
Trial 2 Error Score = _____
Average Error Score = _____

3) **Stance** = Tandem     **Surface** = Firm
Trial 1 Error Score = _____
Trial 2 Error Score = _____
Average Error Score = _____

4) **Stance** = Tandem      **Surface** = Foam
Trial 1 Error Score = _____
Trial 2 Error Score = _____
Average Error Score = _____

5) **Stance** = Single      **Surface** = Firm
Trial 1 Error Score = _____
Trial 2 Error Score = _____
Average Error Score = _____

6) **Stance** = Single      **Surface** = Foam
Trial 1 Error Score = _____
Trial 2 Error Score = _____
Average Error Score = _____


Total BESS Score = _____

**Figure 7.4** Single-leg Romberg stance on a foam surface used with the BESS.

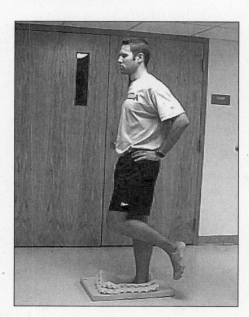

2. Progression across the various phases of balance training involves challenging the diverse systems responsible for maintaining balance and coordination. The clinician needs to start the rehabilitation process with exercises on a static (firm) surface, progressing to semidynamic (foam), dynamic (moving), and sport specific maneuvers. These activities can be conducted using a variety of timing and repetition schemes. Using the tools listed below, perform balance exercises using a variety of stances (double, single, tandem):

- Mini-trampoline
- Rocker board
- Wobble board (BAPS board)
- Perturbations to the shoulder while standing
- Mini-squat maneuver
- Sit-to-stand using a Physioball
- Forward lunges
- Lateral and forward step-ups
- Slant board
- T-band kicks
- Hop drills (diagonal, lateral, forward, bounding)
- Co-contraction drills

Which surfaces created the most difficulty during the balance tasks? Why?

What happens when you closed your eyes?

What stance was the most difficult to maintain? Why?

# Laboratory Exercise 8

# Core Stabilization
# Training in Rehabilitation

## PURPOSE:

Recent advances in rehabilitation have improved the way clinicians treat a variety of injury conditions. While caring for the affected area remains foremost, clinicians have developed interventions to treat the "whole" as well as just the affected "part" of the patient. The purpose of this laboratory task is to introduce the student to the concept of core stability (spinal stability) and to allow ample opportunity to become proficient with the tools, skills, and techniques needed to make this part of your clinical repertoire.

## ATHLETIC TRAINING EDUCATIONAL COMPETENCIES:

*Therapeutic Exercise (Psychomotor Domain)*

- Demonstrates the appropriate application of contemporary therapeutic exercises including the following:

- Exercises to improve neuromuscular coordination and proprioception
- Functional rehabilitation and reconditioning

- Demonstrates the proper techniques for the performance of commonly prescribed rehabilitation and reconditioning exercises.

# ATHLETIC TRAINING CLINICAL PROFICIENCIES:

*Therapeutic Exercise (The student will demonstrate the ability to perform therapeutic exercises.)*

- Exercise to improve neuromuscular control and coordination. The student will demonstrate the ability to instruct the following activities:

### Trunk:

Stabilization
Postural Correction

# REVIEW OF PRINCIPLES:

The concept of core stabilization is most closely related to rehabilitation of low back maladies. As the concept and techniques have evolved, clinicians are now finding ways to incorporate core stabilization training activities into rehabilitation programs involving injuries other than just the spinal column. The "core" can be thought of as the trunk or torso, with the rib cage denoting the upper third and the hip/pelvis region defining the lower third. Upper extremity movements can be influenced by the rib region, while lower extremity movements can be profoundly affected by the hip/pelvis. Therefore, the mechanical and neuromuscular stability of the core can have an effect on upper and lower extremity function.[1] Pelvic positioning, rib cage positioning, and neuromuscular recruitment of the anterior and posterior trunk musculature must all be included in a complete core-stabilization program.[1] It is important to remember that stabilization training works the core stabilizers in their natural fashion, not as prime movers but as primary stabilizers.[2]

The exercise format for core stabilization emphasizes both muscular strength and endurance, with additional considerations made for proprioception.[2] Postural awareness and correction activities are also part of the fundamental process. Typically, strength exercises are introduced and then followed by more advanced endurance and proprioception activities. Initial movements are deliberate and natural, while more sport-specific, higher intensity functional activities are instituted later. Bandy and Sanders [2] suggest that the clinician consider the following basic principles when beginning a training progression:

(1) Monitor the effects of weight bearing

(2) Use stable before unstable postures

(3) Use simple motions before combined movements

(4) Integrate gross motions before isolated, fine motor patterns

A variety of exercise activities and rehabilitation tools can be adapted to fit the needs of the patient with one's creative imagination being the only limitation. It is suggested that all core-stabilization routines be administered following a generalized warm-up that includes both flexibility and cardiovascular components.

## TEXTBOOK REFERENCE CHAPTER:

Chapter 10

## REFERENCES:

1. King, M.A. 2000. Core stability: Creating a foundation for functional rehabilitation. *Athletic Therapy Today* 5(2):6-13.

2. Bandy, W.D., and B. Sanders. 2001. *Therapeutic Exercise: Techniques for Intervention.* Philadelphia, PA: Lippincott Williams & Wilkins.

## LABORATORY EXERCISES:

1. Students must begin core stabilization exercises from the neutral or functional position of the spine. Having an understanding of this position is essential so that they can instruct their patients in finding this position from which all stabilization exercises should begin. Working alone and lying on the treatment table, position yourself into lumbopelvic neutral. Envision your naval as 12:00 o'clock and pubic bone as 6:00 o'clock. You should then rock back and forth slowly between these two points. Locate the point within this range that is most comfortable for you and use this to define your "neutral" point. Next, you should work with your partner as if they were a patient and instruct them how they should locate the lumbopelvic neutral position.

King[1] describes an alternative method using a foam roller for tactile feedback. Lie lengthwise on the foam roller and posteriorly tilt the pelvis so that the low back just contacts the foam roller (Figure 8.1). The athlete may roll from side-to-side on the roller to help relax the musculature. The patient is then instructed to memorize this position through repeated trials, eventually getting efficient enough so that it can be performed without the arms used for support and in the absence of any excessive foot pressure. Practice this routine, first alone and then with your lab partner.

**Figure 8.1** Lumbopelvic neutral position on a foam roller.

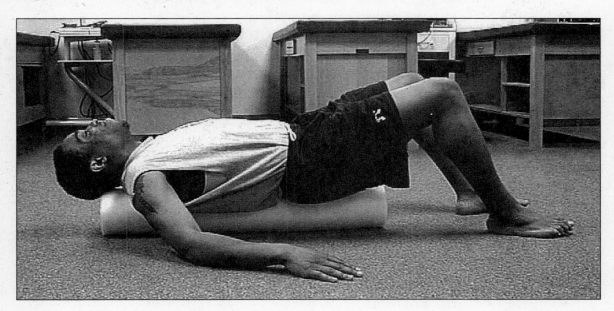

2.  Having developed an understanding of lumbopelvic "neutral", it is now time to advance to more challenging core stabilization exercises.  Keep in mind that a number of rehabilitation tools can be utilized in the performance of the stabilization routines including, but not limited to:

- Foam rollers
- Stability balls
- Free weights
- Elastic bands
- Wobble boards
- Sliding boards

Students should be able to incorporate core stabilization routines that focus on the (1) lower core, (2) upper core, and (3) posterior core (back/trunk extensors). Working in pairs, experiment with the following core-stabilization exercises both on yourself and via instruction with your lab partner. (Keep in mind that some of the exercises listed below may have other names associated with them.)

- Unilateral straight leg lift/raise
- "Dying Bug" exercise position
- Bridge position with variations (side-bridge, shoulder bridge, etc...)
- Unilateral straight leg lift/raise in bridge position
- Prone straight leg raise (hip extension)
- Quadruped position with and without extremity lifts (multifidi or "Bird-dog" position)
- Kneeling with thoracic rotation
- Quadruped position with foam rollers
- Balance board in prone position
- Sliding board in prone position
- Single leg knee-to-chest exercise
- 90° hip flexion/90° knee flexion position while supine
- Superman (flying) positions
- Bridging with the stability ball (including extremity lifts)
- Scapular retraction with knees flexed and extended on therapeutic ball
- Gluteal-abdominal hold with stability ball
- The bicycle position
- "Fire hydrant" position

Students should be able to perform these exercises using a variety of duration, repetition, and set schemes. The complexity of each exercise can be challenged by adding resistance along with either upper or lower extremity functional movements as your patient becomes more proficient and experienced with the routines.

# *Laboratory Exercise 9*

# Reactive Neuromuscular Training (Plyometrics) in Rehabilitation

## PURPOSE:

The ability to jump and land effectively are critical components in a variety of athletic endeavors. With this in mind, clinicians have used jump training (plyometrics) as a facet of countless rehabilitation programs with a variety of patients (athletes) regardless of what sport they play. The purpose of this laboratory exercise is to review the foundational aspects of plyometric training and to involve the student in a number of activities that they will find useful in the implementation of these skills in a rehabilitation setting.

## ATHLETIC TRAINING EDUCATIONAL COMPETENCIES:

*Risk Management and Injury Prevention (Psychomotor Domain)*

- Implements and administers fitness programs, including correction or modification of inappropriate, unsafe, or dangerous fitness routines.

*Therapeutic Exercise (Psychomotor Domain)*

- Demonstrates the appropriate application of contemporary therapeutic exercises including the following:

- Plyometrics-dynamic reactive exercise
- Functional rehabilitation and reconditioning

- Demonstrates the proper techniques for the performance of commonly prescribed rehabilitation and reconditioning exercises.

## ATHLETIC TRAINING CLINICAL PROFICIENCIES:

*Therapeutic Exercise (The student will demonstrate the ability to perform therapeutic exercises.)*

- Exercise to improve muscular speed

### Upper & Lower Body:

Reaction Drills

- Exercise to improve muscular power

- The student will demonstrate the ability to instruct plyometric exercises for the upper and lower extremities.

## REVIEW OF PRINCIPLES:

Jump training has its roots in Eastern Europe. For many years the Eastern Bloc countries used this training method to train athletes involved in sports requiring explosive muscular movements (weight lifting, track and field, etc...) It was first introduced in this country in the early 70's and used predominately as a training technique for track and field athletes. It has since become a common entity of most strength and conditioning programs across the land. It has even found a place in athletic injury rehabilitation.

Power is a product of both strength and speed. Plyometric or reactive neuromuscular training is intended to get at the core of both components in an attempt to improve athletic performance in events requiring explosive power. The physiological basis for plyometric training lies in the fact that muscles have a natural tendency to rebound when stretched rapidly.[1] The ability for the muscle(s) to react (contract) following a stretch is similar to taking a rubber-band and stretching it to be flown across the room, the greater you stretch it, the further it will fly. In the muscle, an eccentric muscle action is utilized to pre-load (stretch) the muscle so that the antagonistic concentric muscle action can be enhanced, resulting in a greater jump. The reversal of muscle actions is known as the amortization phase of the stretch-shortening cycle.[1] Simply put, you're able to jump higher following landing from a jump or step-down, than you are if you just jump from a standing position.

Stretch-shortening cycles of muscles are inherent to sport. There are three phases of the stretch-shortening cycle (SSC): eccentric phase, amortization phase, and the concentric phase. For an exercise to be truly plyometric, it must be a movement preceded by an eccentric muscle action.[2] This results not only in stimulating the proprioceptors sensitive to rapid stretch (muscle spindles), but also in loading the serial elastic components (tendons and cross-bridges in the muscle fibers) with a tension force from which they can rebound.[2] There are a number of quality multimedia resources available for the student to learn in greater detail the physiological, biomechanical, and clinical applicability of plyometrics if they so choose.

Plyometric training in a rehabilitation setting is typically sport-specific. Before plyometric activities are initiated into a rehabilitation plan it is imperative that the patient (athlete) meet the biomechanical, stability, coordination, and flexibility prerequisites to safely and effectively perform the skilled maneuvers. The clinician should pre-screen the athletes in an attempt to determine their qualifications for getting involved in such explosive endeavors. Traditional plyometric routines were developed for the lower extremity; however many of the routines, principles, and equipment can be modified to enable incorporation into upper extremity programs too. The clinician should be aware of the demands plyometric training places on the body and therefore make considerations for intensity, volume, duration, frequency, and recovery time when designing and implementing such programs.

## TEXTBOOK REFERENCE CHAPTER:

Chapter 11

## REFERENCES:

1. Chu, D.A. 1999. Plyometrics in sports injury rehabilitation and training. *Athletic Therapy Today* 4(3):7-11.

2. Chu, D.A. 1992. *Jumping into Plyometrics.* Champaign, IL: Leisure Press, A Division of Human Kinetics Publishers, Inc.

3. Swanik, C.B., and K.A. Swanik. 1999. Plyometrics in rehabilitating the lower extremity. *Athletic Therapy Today* 4(3):16-22.

4. Courson, R., M.Dillon, T. Hicks, L. Navitskis, and M. Ferrara. 1999. Plyometrics in rehabilitation of the upper extremity. *Athletic Therapy Today* 4(3):25-29.

# LABORATORY EXERCISES:

1. Vertical jump performance is a basic measure of power. The vertical jump maneuver can be performed in a variety of ways. It can also be performed with and without arm movements. Using either a commercial vertical jump testing device (ex. Vertec™ --- see pg.51) or the side wall with chalk technique, execute the following jumps:

- Jump from a standing position without bending your knees
- Jump from a position of approximately 45° of knee flexion
- Jump from a position of full knee flexion (squat position)
- Perform the jump after bending down to 45° of knee flexion from a standing position and immediately executing the vertical jump
- Perform the jump after bending down to full knee flexion (squat position) from a standing position and immediately executing the vertical jump
- Perform the jump after stepping down and landing on both feet from a boxes ranging in height from 6" to 24" and immediately executing the vertical jump

Perform three (3) jumps for each taking the average jump height (inches or centimeters) and comparing across the different performances. (Refer to laboratory exercise #4 in Chapter 6 for more detail on vertical jump measurements)

| Jump Condition | Jump #1 | Jump #2 | Jump #3 | Average |
|---|---|---|---|---|
| Standing - no arms | | | | |
| Standing - rocking arms | | | | |
| Knees bent to 45° - no arms | | | | |
| Knees bent to 45° - rocking arms | | | | |
| Begin standing – bend to 45° of knee flexion – rocking arms | | | | |
| Knees bent fully - no arms | | | | |

| | | | |
|---|---|---|---|
| Knees bent fully - rocking arms | | | |
| Begin standing – bend to full knee flexion – rocking arms | | | |
| Begin standing – jump down from 6" box height – rocking arms | | | |
| Begin standing – jump down from 12" box height – rocking arms | | | |
| Begin standing – jump down from 18" box height – rocking arms | | | |
| Begin standing – jump down from 24" box height – rocking arms | | | |

You should begin to see differences in heights according to the various routines you perform.

Which combination of skill components leads to the highest jump heights? Why?

Which combination of skill components leads to the lowest jump heights? Why?

2. Well known plyometric guru Dr. Donald Chu has developed six (6) classifications of lower extremity plyometric exercises [2]:

- Jumps-in-place
- Standing jumps
- Multiple hops and jumps
- Bounding
- Box drills
- Depth jumps

Working in groups of two, instruct your lab partner to execute each of these basic jumps (Reprinted by permission from D.A. Chu, 1998, *Jumping into plyometrics*, 2nd ed., Champaign, IL:  Human Kinetics Publishers, pp. 82, 86, 95, 114, & 123.)

a) **Figure 9.1**  Tuck-jump

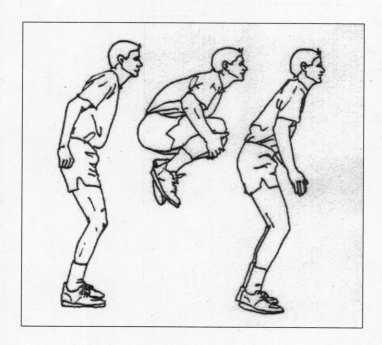

b) **Figure 9.2**  Standing long-jump

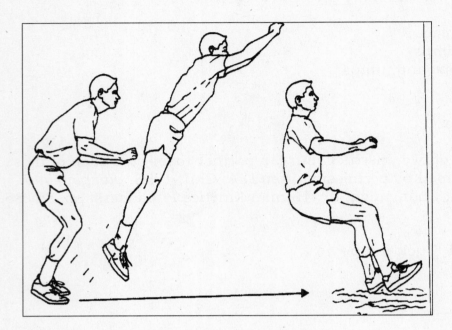

c) **Figure 9.3**  Diagonal cone-hops

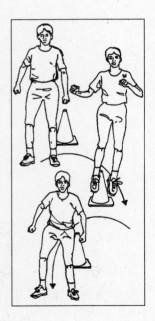

d) **Figure 9.4** Squat depth jumps

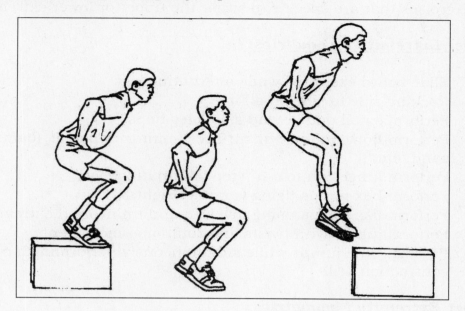

e) **Figure 9.5** Power skipping

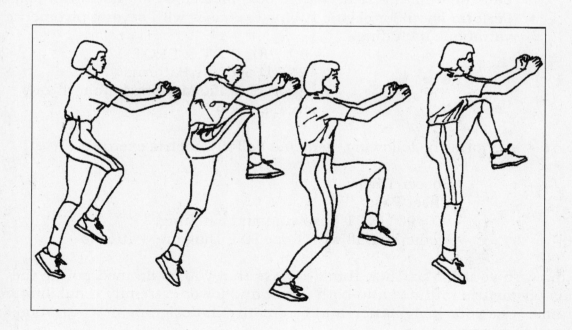

After completing these basic jumps, instruct your partner in performing the following exercises that are specific to either the upper or lower extremity:

### _Lower Extremity Plyometrics:_ [3]

- Slide board exercises while alternating legs
- Rocking side to side on a Fitter
- Perform small double and single leg hops
- Perform hops on uneven surfaces (mini-trampoline, foam mat, sand, etc...)
- Perform lunges on to a 6" step (alternating legs)
- Perform box jumps using various heights
- Perform box jumps using involved and uninvolved extremity only
- Perform jumps with twists and rotational movements
- Perform cone jumps while simultaneously performing a co-contraction drill

### _Upper Extremity Plyometrics:_ [4]

- Perform plyometric push-ups with several variations (wall, incline, ballistic wall, hip sled, double box, medicine ball, mini-trampoline)
- Perform shoulder elastic tubing exercises with several plyometric variations including:
  - 90°/90° IROT & EROT
  - PNF Diagonals Patterns
  - Sport Specific Motions (pitch, throw, serve, stroke)

- Perform the following medicine ball plyometric exercises:

  - Soccer Throw
  - Chest Pass
  - 90°/90° IROT (throwing and catching)
  - Medicine Ball with Rope PNF Diagonal Patterns

Working with your lab partner, think of ways that you could incorporate the various plyometric routines into both upper and lower extremity rehabilitation programs. Use your imagination and be creative in designing new variations to these existing routines.

# *Laboratory Exercise 10*

# Open-versus Closed-Kinetic-Chain Exercise in Rehabilitation

## PURPOSE:

The majority of exercises incorporated into rehabilitation programs consist of both open- (OKC) and closed-kinetic chain (CKC) routines. Historically, OKC assessment and rehabilitation exercises were popular in the 1980's, while CKC routines seemed to have dominated the rehabilitation circles in the 1990's. Perhaps, the integration of both types of exercise programs is the best approach for the well-being and success of your patient. The purpose of this laboratory exercise is to review the concepts and theory behind OKC and CKC exercises and familiarize the student with some well accepted routines that can be incorporated into most, if not all, rehabilitation programs. It is important to remember that most of the information gleaned from this lab can be modified and used with rehab programs/tools described elsewhere in this lab manual.

## ATHLETIC TRAINING EDUCATIONAL COMPETENCIES:

*Risk Management and Injury Prevention (Psychomotor Domain)*

- Implements and administers fitness programs, including correction or modification of inappropriate, unsafe, or dangerous fitness routines.

*Therapeutic Exercise (Psychomotor Domain)*

- Demonstrates the appropriate application of contemporary therapeutic exercises including the following:

- Open- versus closed-kinematic chain exercise
- Functional rehabilitation and reconditioning

- Demonstrates the proper techniques for the performance of commonly prescribed rehabilitation and reconditioning exercises.

## ATHLETIC TRAINING CLINICAL PROFICIENCIES:

*Therapeutic Exercise (The student will demonstrate the ability to perform therapeutic exercises.)*

- Exercise to improve muscular strength, endurance, speed, and power.

## REVIEW OF PRINCIPLES:

The concept of the kinetic chain originated in the mechanical engineering literature in the late 1800's. The notion was later adapted to fit human movement theory and presented by Steindler in 1955.[1] For purposes of our discussion we will define OKC and CKC exercise using definitions adopted from Ellenbecker and Davies.[2] An OKC exercise or movement pattern is one where the distal aspect of the extremity is not fixed to an object and terminates free in space. A CKC exercise or movement is one where the distal aspect of the extremity is fixed to an object that is either stationary or moving. The characteristics of both OKC and CKC exercises are nicely summarized in the following table

**Table 10.1** Characteristics of OKC and CKC activities. (Reprinted by permission from Ellenbecker and Davies [2]):

| Characteristic | OKC | CKC |
|---|---|---|
| Stress Pattern | Rotary | Linear |
| Number of joint axes | One primary | Multiple |
| Nature of joint segments | One stationary, the other mobile | Both segments move simultaneously |
| Number of moving joints | Isolated joint motion | Multiple-joint motion |
| Planes of movement | One (single) | Multiple (triplanar) |
| Muscular involvement | Isolation of muscle or muscle groups, minimal muscular co-contraction | Significant muscular co-contraction |
| Movement pattern | Often non-functional movement patterns | Significant functionally oriented movement patterns |

Biomechanically and physiologically, OKC and CKC exercises are different. It is important that the student review these principles for a greater understanding before utilizing the exercise routines in a clinical setting. Open- and closed-kinetic chain exercises have many distinct advantages and disadvantages, yet can both be utilized to assist the clinician in offering a safe and effective rehabilitation plan. Interestingly, there is some evidence suggesting a positive correlation between OKC testing and functional performance, despite what some critics fault OKC exercises as being non-functional.[3] The decision as to whether or not OKC vs. CKC exercises are used should be done at the discretion of the clinician and the intended treatment goals.

Historically, CKC exercise routines were directed toward the lower extremity. However, in recent years clinicians have been able to adopt them to the upper extremity as well. Traditionally, OKC exercise interventions have been performed utilizing isokinetic dynamometry. Because we have devoted a later chapter in this manual to isokinetics, the focus of this laboratory will be on CKC exercises for both the upper and lower extremity.

## TEXTBOOK REFERENCE CHAPTER:

Chapter 12

## REFERENCES:

1. Steindler, A. 1955. *Kinesiology of the Human Body*. Springfield, IL: Charles C. Thomas Publishers.

2. Ellenbecker, T.S., and G.J. Davies. 2001. *Closed-Kinetic Chain Exercise*. Champaign, IL: Human Kinetics.

3. Davies, G.J. 1995. The need for critical thinking in rehabilitation. *Journal of Sport Rehabilitation*. 4(1):1-22.

4. Davies, G.J., and D.A. Zillmer. 2000. Functional progression of exercise during rehabilitation. In: *Knee Ligament Rehabilitation, 2nd Edition*. Philadelphia, PA: Churchill Livingstone.

5. Davies, G.J., and S. Dickoff-Hoffman. 1993. Neuromuscular testing and rehabilitation of the shoulder complex. *Journal of Orthopedic and Sport Physical Therapy.* 18(2):449-458.

## LABORATORY EXERCISES:

1. In order for clinicians to select appropriate OKC or CKC exercises for use in the rehabilitation plan they need to be able to assess the functional abilities of their patients. Ellenbecker and Davies have labeled this as the "Functional Testing Algorithm for OKC and CKC Activities".[2] In this lab exercise we will use selected portions of the testing battery so that the student can become familiar with some of the functional test scores needed to make an informed and confident decision about advancing through a CKC rehabilitation protocol. The following tests have been excerpted from their testing algorithm:

a) Functional Jump Test [4]

The two-legged functional jump test measures bilateral lower-leg power. The test is performed with the hands held behind the back in order to minimize compensatory movements from the trunk and limbs (Figure 10.1).

**Figure 10.1** Starting position for the Functional Jump test.

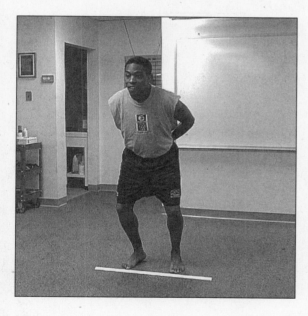

Four (4) graded warm-up jumps are performed at 25%, 50%, 75% and 100% of maximum. The average of three (3) maximum jump efforts normalized as a percentage of the persons total height is used to determine ability to perform CKC exercise.  Percentages (distance as a % of height) ranging from 90% - 100% for males and 80% - 100% for females are acceptable and warrant progression to the next testing sequence.

**Functional Jump Test Scoring Template:**

*Jump #1 Distance* = _____ cm

*Jump #2 Distance* = _____ cm

*Jump #3 Distance* = _____ cm

*Average Jump Distance* = _____ cm

*Average Jump Distance/Height in cm* = _____

*Percentage Value* = _____

*Acceptable* _____          *Unacceptable* _____

b) <u>Functional Hop Test</u> [4]

This test is performed in a similar manner to the two-legged jump, except that it requires taking off and landing on one leg (involved vs. uninvolved) (Figure 10.2). Bilateral comparisons are made and progression allowed if males fall within 80% - 100% and females fall between 70% and 100% (distance as a % of height). It is important to look for any hesitation, limping, angulation, or other body movements that may indicate that the patient is not quite ready for this phase of functional progression.

**Figure 10.2** Starting position for the Functional Hop test.

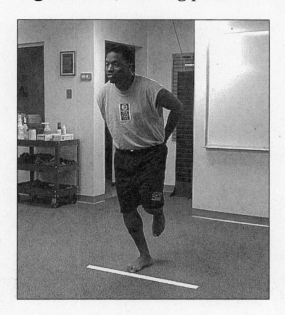

**Uninvolved Extremity**

*Jump #1 Distance =* _____ cm

*Jump #2 Distance =* _____ cm

*Jump #3 Distance =* _____ cm

*Average Jump Distance =* _____ cm

*Average Jump Distance/Height in cm =* _____

*Percentage Value =* _____

*Acceptable* _____      *Unacceptable* _____

## Involved Extremity

*Jump #1 Distance =* _____ cm

*Jump #2 Distance =* _____ cm

*Jump #3 Distance =* _____ cm

*Average Jump Distance =* _____ cm

*Average Jump Distance/Height in cm =* _____

*Percentage Value =* _____

*Acceptable* _____      *Unacceptable* _____

The push-up has for many years been the assessment tool of choice for determining upper extremity CKC readiness. In 1993 Davies and Dickoff-Hoffman developed a modification they called the "CKC Upper Extremity Stability Test".[5]

c) CKC Upper Extremity Stability Test [5]

The test is performed in the push-up position (males) or modified push-up position on knees (females) between two markings that are three (3) feet apart (Figure 10.3).

**Figure 10.3** CKC Upper Extremity Stability test starting position.

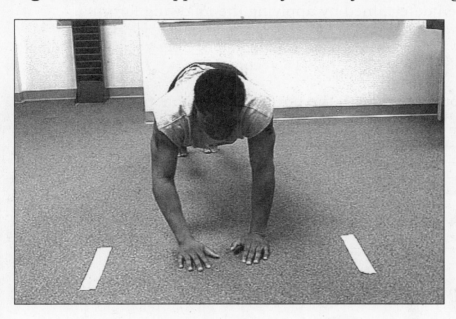

The subject moves their hands back and forth (criss – cross fashion) from each line marking as many times as possible in 15 seconds (Figure 10.4). The number of lines touched with each hand is then totaled. Begin with one sub-maximal warm-up trial, followed by three (3) test trials. The average of the three (3) trials is then used as the final score value.

Scores are then normalized for body height (cm).

$$Score = \frac{\text{\# of lines touched}}{\text{Height (in)}}$$

Power is then determined by applying the following formula:

$$Power = \frac{68\% \text{ body weight X \# of lines touched}}{15 \text{ seconds}}$$

Compare your scores with the norms in the table provided below:

| Norm | Male (Average) | Female (Average) |
|---|---|---|
| Touches | 14.5 | 20.5 |
| Power | 150 | 135 |
| Score | .26 | .31 |

**Figure 10.4** Proper execution of the CKC Upper Extremity Stability test

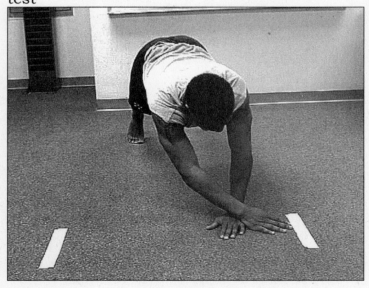

2. There are a number of upper and lower extremity CKC exercises that a student should be familiar with in a clinical environment. The determination of when to use these exercises is left up to the discretion of the individual clinician based on how they can help accomplish the rehabilitation goals. The following is a compendium of CKC exercises commonly used in rehab programs. The student should practice each of these techniques to gain the confidence and skill necessary to employ them in a clinical setting. The student should be aware that there may be more than one name for some of these exercises based on regional and cultural differences. The student is directed to their textbook or one of the references listed for further clarification on execution of these maneuvers.

### Upper Extremity Exercises:

- Weight shifting/Rhythmic stabilization/Perturbation training (standing, quadruped, tripod, biped)
- Weight shifting (BAPS board, wobble board, KAT system, Plyoball)
- Push-ups (Plyoball, stair-climber, Shuttle, with a plus, wall)
- Single-arm lateral steps-ups
- Press-ups
- Slide board exercises ("wax on – wax off" routine)
- Joint approximation with stability ball
- Wheelbarrow walks
- Upper-body treadmill walking

### Lower Extremity Exercises:

- Mini-squats
- Wall slides
- Lunges
- Leg press
- Stair climbing
- Lateral step-ups
- Standing TKE's with rubber tubing
- Stationary cycling
- Mini-trampoline
- Slide board exercises
- Tubing exercises (tubing walk, step-ups/downs with resistance, forward running, retro running, co-contraction drills)

- VersaClimber
- Plyometric box jumps
- Fastex computerized functional training
- Balance boards
- Foam rollers
- Elliptical running machine
- Agility, carioca, cutting, jump-stop drills

# *Laboratory Exercise 11*

# Isokinetics in Rehabilitation

## PURPOSE:

The popularity of isokinetic exercise and evaluation in the clinical environment reached its peak in the mid-1980's. Despite its fleeting moment of glory, isokinetic assessments remain the standard for strength evaluations in clinical settings today. It is vital that clinical education exposes students to the concepts, principles, and techniques of isokinetic dynamometry so that they can become competent professionals when called upon to involve this tool in the rehabilitation environment. Therefore, the purpose of this laboratory task is to review with the student the foundational aspects that govern isokinetic exercise and to afford the student an opportunity to become proficient with performing isokinetic assessments in the laboratory setting.

## ATHLETIC TRAINING EDUCATIONAL COMPETENCIES:

*Risk Management and Injury Prevention (Psychomotor Domain)*

- Performs appropriate tests and examinations for pre-participation physical exam as required by the appropriate governing agency and or physician. (this may include an isokinetic strength assessment)

- Able to operate contemporary isometric, isotonic, and isokinetic strength testing devices.

- Implements and administers fitness programs, including correction or modification of inappropriate, unsafe, or dangerous fitness routines.

*Therapeutic Exercise (Psychomotor Domain)*

- Demonstrates the appropriate application of contemporary therapeutic exercises including the following:

- Isometric, isotonic, and isokinetic exercise
- Eccentric vs. concentric exercise
- Open- versus closed-kinematic chain exercise

- Demonstrates the proper techniques for the performance of commonly prescribed rehabilitation and reconditioning exercises.

- Inspects therapeutic exercise equipment to ensure safe operating condition.

## ATHLETIC TRAINING CLINICAL PROFICIENCIES:

*Risk Management and Injury Prevention (The student will operate and instruct the use of isometric, isotonic, and isokinetic weight training equipment.)*

- The student will demonstrate the ability to perform an isokinetic test for the knee and shoulder.

- The student will demonstrate the ability to interpret data obtained from isokinetic testing and to use this information to determine appropriate follow-up care.

*Therapeutic Exercise (The student will demonstrate the ability to perform therapeutic exercises.)*

- Exercise to improve muscular strength, endurance, speed, and power.

## REVIEW OF PRINCIPLES:

Hislop and Perrine were the first to introduce the concept of isokinetic assessment in a clinical and research environment.[1]  Isokinetics are now well-accepted world-wide as the standard for strength measurement in a clinical setting.  Isokinetic strength assessments have been thoroughly researched through the years and the measurements have been shown to be both reliable and valid.  Isokinetic theory focuses on exercise that is performed at a fixed speed (velocity) with an accommodating or variable resistance. To be considered truly isokinetic, the exercise or test repetition sequence must be performed with maximal effort throughout the range of motion. Thus, verbal encouragement and visual feedback used as reinforcement tools are a necessary and vital component of isokinetic performance.

Contemporary isokinetic dynamometers are interfaced with sophisticated computer systems enabling the clinician to effectively conduct an isokinetic evaluation with ease. Additionally, the dynamometers are versatile enough so that they can be utilized for a variety of exercise routines including isometric, isotonic, and isokinetic applications. In order for the clinician to conduct a safe and proper isokinetic assessment they must first consider a number of factors that are relevant to a valid and reliable test. These factors include:

- Force vs. torque measurement
- Velocity/speed and considerations for specificity
- Active vs. passive mode
- Eccentric vs. concentric mode
- Range of motion
- Gravity correction
- Patient positioning and stabilization
- Pre-loading
- Test vs. exercise protocols
- Data output and interpretation
- Agonist vs. antagonist ratios and muscular imbalances
- Force-velocity relationships (FVR's)

Although isokinetic equipment is expensive to purchase, isokinetic exercise has several advantages to offer over isometric and isotonic activities. These advantages include: [2]

- Permits isolation of weak muscle groups
- Accommodating resistance provides maximal resistance throughout the exercised range of motion
- Accommodating resistance provides inherent safety mechanism
- Permits quantification of torque, work, and power

There are only a few manufacturers of isokinetic dynamometers left today. However, due in part to the dependability and durability of those dynamometers previously made, several different dynamometers are still in use. The following table was revised from that presented in the book "Principles and Practice of Isokinetics in Sports Medicine and Rehabilitation" and lists some of the more common dynamometers and their features.[3]

**Table 11.1** List of common isokinetic dynamometers.

| Type | Models | Modes* | Speed Spectrum |
|------|--------|--------|----------------|
| Kin Com | 500H, 125e+, 125AP | CON, ECC, CPM, ISOM | 1° - 250° |
| Cybex | II+, 340, 350, 6000, NORM | CON, ECC, CPM, ISOM | 1° - 450° = CON<br>1° - 120° = ECC |
| Biodex | 2000, Multi-Joint System 3 Pro | CON, ECC, CPM, ISOM | 1° - 500° = CON<br>1° - 300° = ECC |
| Lido | Active MJ | CON, ECC, CPM, ISOM | 1° - 400° = CON<br>1° - 250° = ECC<br>1° - 180° = CPM |

*CON = concentric, ECC = eccentric, CPM = continuous passive motion, ISOM = isometric

Students are encouraged to access the internet for more information about the newer isokinetic dynamometers and equipment available today.

## TEXTBOOK REFERENCE CHAPTER:

Chapter 13

## REFERENCES:

1. Hislop, H., and H. Perrine. 1967. The isokinetic concept of exercise. *Physical Therapy* 47:116-125.

2. Perrin, D.H. 1993. *Isokinetic Exercise and Assessment.* Champaign, IL: Human Kinetics Publishers.

3. Chan, K.M., and Maffulli, N. Chief Editors. 1996. *Principles and Practice of Isokinetics in Sports Medicine and Rehabilitation.* Hong Kong: Williams & Wilkens Asia-Pacific Ltd.

4. Oman, J. 2003. Isokinetics in rehabilitation. In *Rehabilitation Techniques in Sports Medicine,* 4th ed. St. Louis, MO: WCB/McGraw-Hill.

## LABORATORY EXERCISES:

1. Select a partner and perform an isokinetic evaluation for both the knee (Figure 11.1) and shoulder (Figure 11.2) joints.

**Figure 11.1** Isokinetic Testing for the Knee Joint (FLEX/EXT).

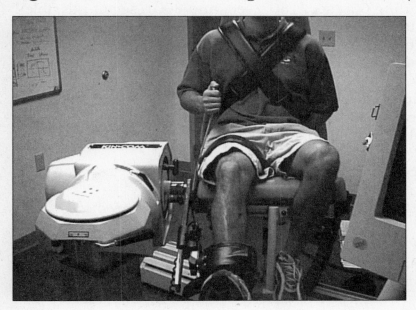

**Figure 11.2** Isokinetic Testing for the Shoulder Joint (IROT/EROT).

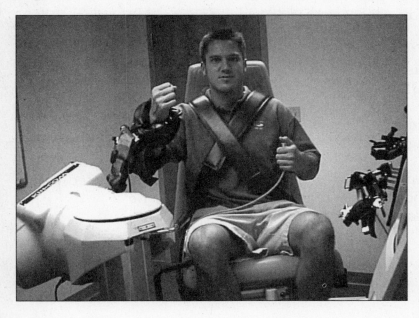

You are instructed to refer to the manufacturers' operations manual for the specifics of each setup. Assess isokinetic strength of the knee flexors (hamstrings) and extensors (quadriceps) both eccentrically (ECC) and concentrically (CON), while for the shoulder joint assess strength of the internal (IROT) and external rotators (EROT). Perform the evaluation at a variety of test velocities including 60°/sec, 180°/sec, and 300°/sec (if possible). Pay particular attention to stabilization of the trunk and limb to be tested. Have your partner perform the test repetitions with and without verbal encouragement and visual feedback. Be certain to allow enough practice/warm-up especially with the ECC repetitions. Eccentric repetitions tend to be somewhat novel and may require some practice on the part of the patient to become accustomed to performing. Print out a copy of the isokinetic evaluation performed on each joint and answer the following questions:

a) Which muscle group was stronger in each assessment?

b) At what speed was the greatest amount of torque/force produced?

c) What are the units for torque and force? (Students should be able to interpret the results in both metric and imperial/US systems.)

d) Compare force production at each velocity. Is ECC or CON force production higher? Why?

e) Was gravity correction necessary for either of these test positions? If yes, why?

f) What commands (push, pull, hold, etc...) did you use when the subject was performing the CON vs. ECC portion of the evaluation?

g) What effect if any did visual feedback and verbal encouragement have on the isokinetic strength performance?

h) What are some potential sources of error that may be associated with the repeatability/reproducibility/reliability of the isokinetic measurements you attained today?

2. Isokinetic dynamometry can provide for an excellent study of force-velocity relationships.  The clinician can use the FVR as a basis for designing a rehabilitation program.[4]  In theory, the FVR consists of two important isokinetic variables that the clinician can utilize:  velocity (speed) and force (torque).  Both of the variables can be plotted together with force on the $y$ axis and velocity on the $x$ axis. (Students should refer to a kinesiology or biomechanics textbook for further information on FVR).  A plot of the FVR for knee extension strength offers valuable insight into this traditional relationship.

Perform a velocity spectrum strength assessment of your lab partner's quadriceps (knee extension) strength.  Use a wide array of velocities including 0°/sec (isometric hold), 30°/sec, 60°/sec, 90°/sec, 120°/sec, 150°/sec, and 180°/sec.  You will need to have both CON and ECC force production at each velocity.  Perform three (3) maximal test repetitions at each speed.  Be certain that you give approximately one (1) minute of rest in between each different velocity presentation.  Print out a copy of the evaluation and use the following template for recording the average peak torque measurement at each velocity:

| Speed/Velocity | CON Peak Torque | ECC Peak Torque |
| --- | --- | --- |
| 0°/sec | | |
| 30°/sec | | |
| 60°/sec | | |
| 90°/sec | | |
| 120°/sec | | |
| 150°/sec | | |
| 180°/sec | | |

Upon completing the measurements, plot out your force-velocity curve using a piece of graph paper or a computer software program such as Microsoft Excel.  On the $x$ axis (velocity) "0" should represent the isometric point with CON measurements to the right of that point (positive direction) and the ECC measurements to the left of that point (negative direction).  Based on your graph answer the following questions:

a) What is the shape of your CON curve, ECC curve?

b) What is the physiological basis that you can use to explain the differences in CON vs. ECC force production across the velocities tested?

c) Is your isometric force production greater than (>), less than (<), or equal (=) to your CON force at 30°/sec? How about your ECC force at 30°/sec?

d) If you were to extrapolate out to points past 180°/sec for both CON and ECC, speculate about what you would see with regards to the curve.

e) Of what use would the FVR be to the clinician? (Consider type of injury, potential force production, dangers associated with ECC exercise modes, etc...)

f) How does your force velocity graph compare to your partner's?

Plot out the FVR for the entire class taking an average of all force values at each velocity and mode (CON vs. ECC).

How does your individual plot compare to the class plot?

How does your class plot compare to the knee extension FVR previously reported in the literature?

3. The muscle groups on both sides of a joint necessarily act reciprocally to produce smooth and coordinated motion.[2] With this in mind, clinicians and physicians often turn to these group comparisons in making rehab progression and return to play decisions. Traditionally, reciprocal muscle group ratios have been calculated comparing CON strength values in the following joints:

- Knee (hamstrings to quadriceps [H:Q ratio])
- Shoulder (abduction to adduction [abd:add ratio] and internal rotators to external rotators [IROT:EROT ratio])
- Ankle (eversion to inversion [E:I ratio])

Newer isokinetic dynamometers allow for a safe and effective means of assessing ECC muscle action and they too can be used in the calculation of reciprocal muscle group ratios.

In this exercise, perform an isokinetic assessment of the knee extensors and flexors along with the shoulder abductors and adductors. The student should be cognizant of stabilization and positioning issues presented previously in this lab. Assess each muscle group at two different velocities both CON and ECC. Extract peak torque data from the computer printout and use these values to calculate your reciprocal muscle group strength ratios. The ratios are easily derived at by dividing the two values according to the ratios listed above. Experiment with several different combinations that will include both motion and muscle action. Remain consistent with your units of measurement (Nm vs. Ft•Lb). The following template can be used to record your measurements for both the right and left extremities:

**Right Side:**

$H_{CON} : Q_{CON} = \rule{3cm}{0.4pt}$

$H_{CON} : Q_{ECC} = \rule{3cm}{0.4pt}$

$H_{ECC} : Q_{CON} = \rule{3cm}{0.4pt}$

$ABD_{CON} : ADD_{CON} = \rule{3cm}{0.4pt}$

$ABD_{CON} : ADD_{ECC} = \rule{3cm}{0.4pt}$

$ABD_{ECC} : ADD_{CON} = \rule{3cm}{0.4pt}$

**Left Side:**

$H_{CON} : Q_{CON} = \rule{3cm}{0.4pt}$

$H_{CON} : Q_{ECC} = \rule{3cm}{0.4pt}$

$H_{ECC} : Q_{CON} = \rule{3cm}{0.4pt}$

$ABD_{CON} : ADD_{CON} = \rule{3cm}{0.4pt}$

$ABD_{CON} : ADD_{ECC} = \rule{3cm}{0.4pt}$

$ABD_{ECC} : ADD_{CON} = \rule{3cm}{0.4pt}$

a) How do your ratios compare to the norms expressed in the literature?

b) How can these ratios be utilized by the clinician to examine muscle imbalances?

c) Can you determine from the ratio which is the stronger of the two muscle groups used?

d) Compare your ratios to those of others in the class. Do you notice any differences between genders? How about differences among body sizes?

e) Why would it be important to utilize the reciprocal muscle action ratios as opposed to examining the ratios form either CON or ECC muscle actions alone? (This will require you to critically think about functional movements --- for example deceleration of the lower leg by the hamstrings acting eccentrically.)

# Laboratory Exercise 12

# Joint Mobilization and Traction Techniques in Rehabilitation

## PURPOSE:

Loss of motion often accompanies joint injury. Typically this loss of motion is associated with pain, tissue contracture, and/or muscle tension. While clinicians have a variety of tools/techniques they may use to improve joint range of motion, perhaps joint mobilization and traction techniques are the most effective. The purpose of this laboratory assignment is to review the foundational concepts of joint mobilization and traction and provide the student with an opportunity to work with and refine their mobilization and traction skills.

## ATHLETIC TRAINING EDUCATIONAL COMPETENCIES:

*Therapeutic Exercise (Psychomotor Domain)*

- Demonstrates the appropriate application of contemporary therapeutic exercises including the following:

- Joint mobilization exercise

- Demonstrates the proper techniques for the performance of commonly prescribed rehabilitation and reconditioning exercises.

# ATHLETIC TRAINING CLINICAL PROFICIENCIES:

*Risk Management and Injury Prevention*

The student will instruct and demonstrate for the client specific flexibility exercises and activities.

- The student will select range-of-motion exercises and activities for all major muscle groups and their associated joints and instruct a client to perform these exercises. The exercises must include the following body regions and joints:

- Cervical region
- Shoulder: joint & girdle
- Elbow
- Wrist
- Hand & fingers
- Lumbar region
- Hip & pelvis
- Knee
- Leg
- Ankle
- Foot & toes

*Therapeutic Exercise (The student will demonstrate the ability to perform therapeutic exercises.)*

- Exercise to improve the range of motion of the upper extremity, lower extremity, trunk, and cervical spine.

- The student will demonstrate the ability to instruct the following exercises:
    - Joint mobilizations
    - Self-mobilizations

- The student will demonstrate the ability to assess joint end point and select and perform appropriate joint mobilization techniques for the appendicular and axial skeleton including the following:

- Long-axis distraction

- Appropriate glides (e.g. anterior/posterior, superior/inferior)

## REVIEW OF PRINCIPLES:

Although we do not always consider it, clinicians utilize joint mobilization techniques often during injury assessment sessions. For example, a valgus/varus stress test or a Lachman test used during the assessment of a knee injury are in actuality versions of joint mobilization techniques. However, the primary aim of joint mobilization is the restoration of normal and pain-free range-of-motion. Specifically, passive movements are applied to joints or soft tissues in a specific manner in order to restore full, free, painless, active ROM. There are a variety of theoretical models in manual therapy including those from such pioneers as Still, Palmer, Cyriax, Kaltenborn, and Maitland.[1] Each model is unique and includes several inconsistencies with the others.

While the clinician can use stretching techniques to improve upon physiological motions, joint mobilization techniques can be performed to improve upon accessory motions. Physiological motions are also referred to as osteokinematic motions and typically occur in the cardinal planes. An example of an osteokinematic motion is flexion/extension movements. Accessory movements, on the other hand, are called arthrokinematic motions; they occur involuntarily and are necessary for full painless ROM.[2] Examples of accessory motions include roll, glide, spin, distraction, and compression. Unlike manipulative movements which include thrusting maneuvers, joint mobilization requires smooth, rhythmic, and low to medium amplitude motions.

Arthrokinematics refers to movements of joint surfaces in relation to one another.[3] The biomechanical principles underlying arthrokinematic motions requires a thorough understanding of the convex and concave rules. In order to understand this concept more effectively, students should envision the knee (tibiofemoral joint) and shoulder (glenohumeral joint) articulations. Additionally, students should work with anatomical models for both of these joints to help them completely understand these difficult concepts. The rule states that when the convex surface is fixed and the concave surface is moving upon it, the arthrokinematics and osteokinematics are in the same direction (i.e. OKC knee flexion). Conversely, when the concave surface is fixed and the convex surface is moving upon it, the arthrokinematics and osteokinematics are in opposite directions (i.e. OKC shoulder flexion). The following diagram illustrates the convex-concave rule for the tibiofemoral articulation (reprinted from Prentice 2003 [3]).

**Figure 12.1** Convex-concave rules applied to the knee joint. **A,** Convex moving on Concave. **B,** Concave moving on Convex.

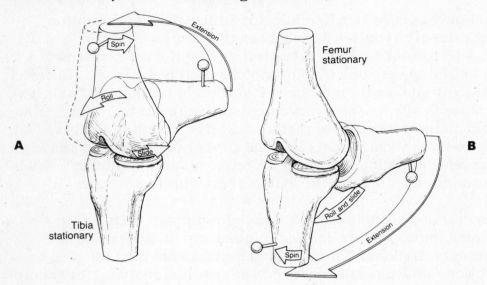

Joint traction techniques are often used in conjunction with joint mobilization by aiding in the inhibition of surrounding musculature. Traction involves pulling on one articulating segment to produce some separation of the two-joint surface.[3] When performed correctly these two techniques can be combined to be a powerful rehabilitation tool to successfully attack conditions of hypomobility.

Success with joint mobilization and traction methods requires consideration for the following:

- Use of sound body mechanics and ergonomics on the part of the clinician
- Work with gravity whenever possible
- Knowledge of "loose or open packed" joint positions
- Mobilization of only one joint surface at a time
- Stabilization of one joint surface
- Mobilization of the other joint surface
- Simultaneous distraction of the joint surfaces
- Knowledge of mobilization grades (reference to Maitland's "Extremity Manipulation" [4])

- Knowledge of contraindications and precautions
- Careful monitoring of the patients pain and evidence of any muscle guarding

## TEXTBOOK REFERENCE CHAPTER:

Chapter 14

## REFERENCES:

1. Holmes, C.F. 2001. Joint mobilization. In *Therapeutic Exercise Techniques for Intervention.* W.D. Bandy and B. Sanders. Baltimore, MD: Lippincott Williams & Wilkins.

2. Kaltenborn, F. 1980. *Mobilization of the extremity joints: Examination and basic treatment techniques.* Norway: Olaf Norlis Bokhandel.

3. Prentice, W. 2003. Joint mobilization and traction techniques in rehabilitation. In *Rehabilitation Techniques in Sports Medicine* 4th ed. St. Louis: WCB McGraw-Hill.

4. Maitland, G. 1977. *Extremity Manipulation.* London: Butterworth.

## LABORATORY EXERCISES:

1. Students wishing to gain an understanding of joint mobilization theory and technique must have a working knowledge of the convex-concave rule and the resting position of the joint to be mobilized. With this in mind complete the following table:

| Joint | Convex Surface | Concave Surface | Resting Position |
|---|---|---|---|
| Sternoclavicular | | | |
| Acromioclavicular | | | |
| Glenohumeral | | | |
| Humeroradial | | | |
| Humeroulnar | | | |
| Radioulnar (proximal) | | | |
| Radioulnar (distal) | | | |
| Radiocarpal | | | |
| Metacarpophalangeal | | | |
| Interphalangeal (hand) | | | |
| Hip | | | |
| Tibiofemoral | | | |

| Joint | Convex Surface | Concave Surface | Resting Position |
|---|---|---|---|
| Patellofemoral | | | |
| Talocrural | | | |
| Subtalar | | | |
| Intertarsal | | | |
| Metatarsophalangeal | | | |
| Interphalangeal (foot) | | | |

2. Taking into consideration the contents of the above-named table, perform *Grade I* (small-amplitude movement at the beginning of the ROM) joint mobilizations to improve the following joint motions on your lab partner. It is imperative that your lab partner is wearing loose fitting clothing including shorts and a T-shirt.

    a) <u>Shoulder Abduction/Flexion</u> (*inferior glide*)

    b) <u>Shoulder EROT/Extension</u> (*anterior glide*)

    c) <u>Shoulder IROT/Flexion</u> (*posterior glide*)

    d) <u>Finger Flexion</u> (*anterior glide*)

    e) <u>Finger Extension</u> (*posterior glide*)

    f) <u>Knee Extension</u> (*anterior glide*)

    g) <u>Knee Flexion</u> (*posterior glide*)

    h) <u>Patellofemoral Motion</u> (*superior & inferior glides*)

    i) <u>Ankle Dorsiflexion</u> (*posterior glide*)

    j) <u>Ankle Plantar Flexion</u> (*anterior glide*)

Once you gain confidence in performing the low-level Grade I mobilizations, choose a few of the motions and attempt to perform some Grade II mobilizations (a large-amplitude movement within the midrange of movement). Students will have an opportunity to experiment with additional joint mobilization and traction techniques as part of the rehabilitation of specific injuries in later chapters in the lab manual.

Answer the following questions as they pertain to the mobilization of the above joint surfaces.

- What problems did you encounter?
- Why is it important to have an understanding of the concept of "end feel"?
- What is the difference between oscillatory vs. thrusting movements?

- What happens when you attempt to perform graded mobilizations in a "closed packed" position?

3. As was mentioned earlier, several joint evaluation techniques are essentially advanced joint mobilization maneuvers.  With this in mind, think of as many assessment techniques (special tests) that could also be thought of as joint mobilization techniques (ex. Lachman test = anterior glide of the tibia on a fixed femur).

| Special Test | Joint | Joint Mobilization Concept (ie. Glide, Roll, Spin, etc..) |
|---|---|---|
|  |  |  |
|  |  |  |
|  |  |  |
|  |  |  |
|  |  |  |
|  |  |  |
|  |  |  |

4. Consider the following scenario and answer the accompanying questions. A quarterback on your football team spent an entire practice throwing footballs in a variety of passing drills. The next day he reports to the clinic with a case of "Frozen Shoulder Syndrome" in his throwing arm. You successfully implement a treatment regime (ICE, e-stim, NSAIDs) for the acute inflammatory process and want to supplement the program with joint mobilizations.

a) What motions will you be concerned with? Why?

b) What grade of mobilization will you use? Why?

c) How much improvement in ROM and pain would you expect to see after one session of joint mobilization?

d) What modalities might you employ following your mobilization session? Why?

e) What things will you consider in making a decision as to when to progress with additional joint mobilization maneuvers?

# *Laboratory Exercise 13*

# PNF and Other Soft Tissue Mobilization Techniques in Rehabilitation

## PURPOSE:

Proprioceptive neuromuscular facilitation (PNF) stretching patterns are a well-theorized and very effective rehabilitation tool. These exercise and stretching patterns, along with several other manual therapy techniques, can complement many rehabilitation protocols and lead to a return to activity on the part of the patient or athlete. The purpose of this laboratory exercise is to provide the student an opportunity to "put into practice" this arsenal of soft tissue mobilization techniques so that they gain the necessary confidence to safely and efficiently use them in a clinical practice setting.

## ATHLETIC TRAINING EDUCATIONAL COMPETENCIES:

*Therapeutic Exercise (Psychomotor Domain)*

- Demonstrates the appropriate application of contemporary therapeutic exercises including the following:

- Proprioceptive neuromuscular facilitation (PNF) for muscular strength/endurance, muscle stretching, and improved range of motion
- Soft tissue mobilization

- Demonstrates the proper techniques for the performance of commonly prescribed rehabilitation and reconditioning exercises.

# ATHLETIC TRAINING CLINICAL PROFICIENCIES:

*Therapeutic Exercise (The student will demonstrate the ability to perform therapeutic exercises.)*

- Exercise to improve neuromuscular control and coordination

  - The student will demonstrate the ability to instruct the following activities:

    - PNF patterns for upper and lower body

# REVIEW OF PRINCIPLES:

Understanding the inflammatory process occurring post-injury is fundamental to rehabilitation interventions. Soft tissue directly affected by the injury and surrounding the involved area will undoubtedly be engaged in the healing process and must prepare itself for the rigors of functional loading. Soft tissue mobilization uses specific, graded, and progressive application of force through the use of physiological, accessory, or combined techniques to promote changes in the viscoelastic response of the tissue in the latter stages of healing.[1] The *Guide to Physical Therapist Practice* defines mobilization as a manual therapy technique comprised of a continuum of skilled passive movements to joints and/or related soft tissues applied at varying speeds and amplitudes and including a small amplitude/high velocity therapeutic movement.[2]

Perhaps the most known and widely used soft tissue mobilization technique is that of proprioceptive neuromuscular facilitation (PNF). As the name implies, joint and soft tissue proprioceptors are stimulated via smooth and functional interaction of both the neurological and muscular systems. PNF activities are a valuable tool in the clinical setting. They restore normal movement patterns, strength, endurance, and ultimately full function.[3] The focus of this review is more on application than theory. Students are encouraged to refer to their textbook for a complete discussion on the physiological basis of PNF interventions.

There is some confusion among clinicians as to the terminology used to describe PNF movement patterns. Terms such as contract-relax, hold-relax, agonist contraction, slow reversal hold-relax, hold-relax with agonist contraction, and contract-relax with agonist contraction add to the confusion. Simply put, a brief contraction before a brief static stretch of the muscle is the mainstay of the PNF techniques used to increase flexibility of the muscle.[4] With the addition of functional diagonal patterns and manual resistance, these same techniques can be utilized to improve muscular strength and endurance. Like any skill, PNF techniques must be practiced in order to be mastered. It is important that students understand the basic principles of PNF so that they will be able to effectively apply the PNF techniques in a clinical setting. The following is a summary of those principles.

- Teach the movement patterns to the patient
- Use mirrors so that the patient can see themselves perform the movements
- Verbal cues are important in successful execution ("push", "pull", "hold", "relax", etc...)
- Tactile pressure aids in guiding the patient through the movements
- The clinician must use good body mechanics and positioning
- Gauge resistance to allow for smooth and coordinated movements
- Rotational movements are a critical component and should be introduced into the patterns
- Work to establish "normal timing" of movements so as to mimic functional activities
- Safely employ "quick stretches" before muscle contractions to facilitate greater muscular involvement

Although PNF activities is the central focus of this laboratory exercise, several other important soft tissue mobilization techniques can be incorporated into the rehabilitation plan. It is crucial that the students have a sound understanding of the theoretical principles that form the foundation of these techniques before employing them in a clinical setting. One traditional osteopathic therapy with some PNF theory involved is muscle energy techniques. Muscle energy is defined as a direct mobilization technique that uses a voluntary contraction by the patient to remedy a soft tissue restriction.[5] Muscle energy techniques have been used to reduce edema, lengthen muscles, strengthen weakened muscles, stretch fascia, and mobilize joints structures. Another closely related soft tissue mobilization technique is called the strain-counterstrain method. The strain-counterstrain technique was first introduced in 1955 by L.H. Jones, a doctor of osteopathic medicine.[6] Other names for this technique include spontaneous release positioning and positional release therapy. The technique is based upon locating tender, painful points in the soft tissues and positioning the patient so that the tenderness is relieved.[7]

Some would argue that sport massage is more of a therapeutic modality than it is a therapeutic exercise. Massage techniques have been employed by clinicians for a variety of ailments; they work to improve flexibility, make pain more tolerable, decrease NM excitability, enhance circulation, and reduce cramping. Therapeutic massage techniques can also be utilized to relieve stress and tension prior to or following competition. Sport massage is usually performed with a specific purpose or goal in mind. Sport massage is traditionally performed on-site in the clinical environment without considerations for privacy being made. The traditional Swedish massage strokes of pétrissage, effleurage, tapotement, and friction, along with sport-specific tissue broadening, are usually administered to athletes. Additional sport-specific massage techniques include friction massage, myofascial release, and acupuncture/trigger point therapies. The following should be given consideration when utilizing sport massage techniques in a rehab setting:

1) Deliver the massage pressure safely through the body to the hands

2) Massage should be performed with a steady and even rhythm

3) Gauge patient response to determine duration

4) In general, the direction of the massage stroke is in-line with the muscle fibers

5) Patient should be in a warm and comfortable position

6) The clinician needs to be cognizant of their own body positioning so that they can perform without undue strain on themselves

7) Sufficient lubricant should be used to allow smooth movement of the hands on the skin

8) Use caution over bony prominences

## TEXTBOOK REFERENCE CHAPTER:

Chapter 15

## REFERENCES:

1. Prentice, W. 2003. PNF and other soft tissue mobilization techniques in rehabilitation. In *Rehabilitation Techniques in Sports Medicine* 4th ed. St. Louis: McGraw-Hill.

2. American Physical Therapy Association (APTA). 2001. *Guide to Physical Therapy Practice* 2nd ed. Alexandria, VA: APTA.

3. Charland, J. 1993. Rehabilitation and PNF. In *Facilitated Stretching* R.E. McAtee. Champaign, IL: Human Kinetics Publishers.

4. Bandy, W.D. 2001. Stretching activities for increasing muscle flexibility. In *Therapeutic Exercise Techniques for Intervention.* Baltimore, MD: Lippincott Williams & Wilkins.

5. Stone, J. 2000. Muscle energy technique. *Athletic Therapy Today.* 5(5):25.

6. Simmons, S.L. Strain and counterstrain technique. DrSimmons.Net Available at: http://pages.prodigy.net/stn1/Counterstrain%20Techniques.htm Accessed December 12, 2002.

7. Stone, J. 2000. Strain-counterstrain. *Athletic Therapy Today.* 5(6):30.

8. Prentice. W. 1993. *Proprioceptive neuromuscular facilitation* [Videotape]. St. Louis, MO: Mosby.

## LABORATORY EXERCISES:

1. In this assignment students will work in groups of two and practice three (3) of the foundational PNF stretching techniques on each other. It is critical that the students work collectively to critique each other so that they both become proficient at hand positioning, manual resistance, and proper cadence. Students are encouraged to refer to their textbook or to view the *Proprioceptive Neuromuscular Facilitation* videotape by Prentice [8] for further instruction on the techniques listed below. Along with your lab partner, practice the following techniques using the hamstring muscle group.

    a) <u>Hold-Relax</u> (Figure 13.1)

Passively flex the hip to full flexion ("relax"). The patient then applies a 10-sec isometric "hold" while attempting to extend the hip (actively contracting the hamstring muscle group) against the resistance of the clinician. Immediately following the "hold", instruct the patient to "relax" and once again passively flex the hip into a greater range of hip flexion. This new stretched position is held for 10-15 sec. Repeat this sequence 3-5 times on each leg. The leg is then lowered following the last stretch.

**Figure 13.1** Athlete being stretched with the "Hold-Relax" PNF technique.

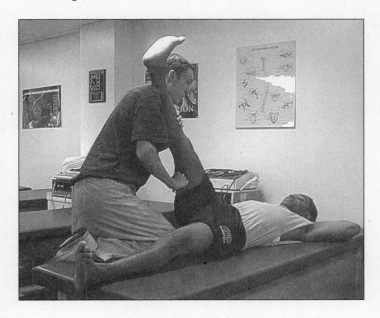

b) <u>Contract-Relax</u> (Figure 13.2)

Passively flex the hip to full flexion ("relax").  Instruct the patient to "contract" the muscles opposite those being stretch (i.e. hip flexors – quadriceps).  By doing so the patient is actively assisting further stretch of the hamstrings.  (It is important that the clinician **does not** assist this movement passively!)  Once the patient has obtained the new stretch position the clinician "holds" the limb for 10-15 sec.  Repeat this sequence 3-5 times on each leg.  The leg is then lowered following the last stretch.

**Figure 13.2**  Athlete being stretched with the "Contract-Relax" PNF technique.

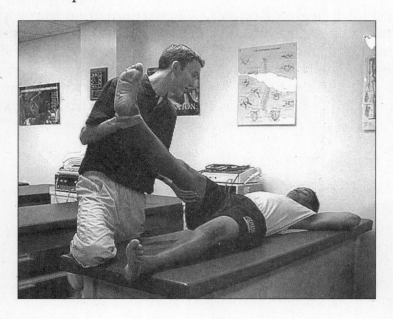

c) <u>Slow Reversal Hold-Relax</u> (Figure 13.3)

Passively flex the hip to full flexion ("relax").  The patient then applies a 10-sec isometric "hold" while attempting to extend the hip (actively contracting the hamstring muscle group) against the resistance of the clinician.  Immediately following the isometric "hold" instruct the patient to "contract" the muscles opposite those being stretch (i.e. hip flexors - quadriceps).  By doing so the patient is actively assisting further stretch of the hamstrings.  (It is important that the clinician **_does not_** assist this movement passively!)  The clinician can now take up any slack in the ROM gained and maintain this position for 10-15 sec.  Repeat this sequence 3-5 times on each leg.  The leg is then lowered following the last stretch.

**Figure 13.3**  Athlete being stretched with the "Slow Reversal Hold-Relax" PNF technique.

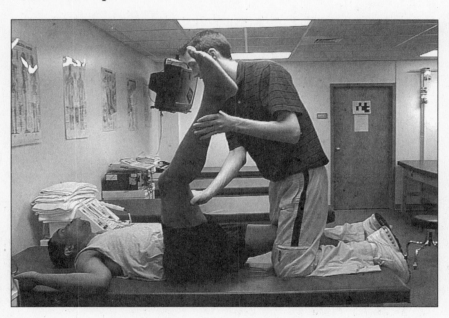

As you become more comfortable and proficient with these techniques, explore ways in which you can apply these PNF stretching techniques to other muscle(s).

- Which technique facilitated the greatest stretch?

- Which technique required the most resistive effort on the part of the clinician?

- Which technique was the most difficult to get the proper cadence sequence?

2. There are many ways PNF stretching and strengthening exercises can be incorporated into a rehabilitation program. This is especially true with throwing athletes (baseball, softball, javelin, shot put). For example baseball pitchers utilize patterns that simulate PNF $D_2$ extension patterns, especially with the delivery of curve balls and sliders. Additionally, deceleration of the arm as it releases the ball follow movements closely resembling PNF $D_1$ and $D_2$ flexion patterns. Furthermore, the scapular stabilizers (rhomboids, traps, levator scapula and serratus anterior) can be rehabilitated using rhythmic stabilization techniques. Each of these techniques can be performed manually by the skilled clinician.

a) Using your knowledge and understanding of the principles of PNF we will now learn the upper extremity diagonal PNF patterns and then incorporate them into both strengthening and stretching routines for the throwing athlete. Both you and your partner should learn and practice the following patterns. (Practice in front of a mirror.) Once you have learned them, try to teach them to your partner.

- $\underline{D_1\ Flexion}$ (flexion-adduction-EROT)

    This is called the "self-feeding" pattern.

- $\underline{D_1\ Extension}$ (extension-abduction-IROT)

    This is often called the "swimmer's stretch".

- $\underline{D_2\ Flexion}$ (flexion-abduction-EROT)

    This patterns mimics "drawing a sword".

- $\underline{D_2\ Extension}$ (extension-adduction-IROT)

    This patterns mimics "sheathing a sword".

b) After you have successfully learned and practiced the diagonal PNF patterns, you are now ready to utilize them to perform a series of stretching and strengthening exercises for the upper extremity. Position your lab partner either supine ($D_1$ Flexion, $D_1$ Extension, $D_2$ Extension) or prone ($D_2$ Flexion) on the treatment plinth and perform the above named stretched (some clinicians may find it necessary to perform $D_2$ Flexion in a supine position).  Stretching should be pain-free.  You may incorporate each of the stretching sequences you practiced in lab exercise #1. Following the completion of the stretching, add manual resistance to each of the four (4) patterns for strengthening purposes.  These same patterns can be used to isolate lower extremity muscle patterns.

c) Based on your experiences in this laboratory and with your own clinical rotations, answer the following questions.

- What upper and lower extremity functional movements mimic the PNF patterns learned in lab?

- Why is it important to stress the rotational component of these maneuvers?

- How could the clinician use PNF activities to improve muscle endurance?

- What routines would you incorporate if asked to develop a supplemental PNF stretching and strengthening routine for a swim team?   Why?  (Consider simplicity and time factors).

3. A good beginning massage stroke for the student to learn and practice is effleurage (Figure 13.4). Get with your lab partner and practice the effleurage stroke technique on the mid-belly of the quadriceps muscle. Position your subject on the treatment table and properly drape the area to be treated with toweling. Use a good, hypo-allergenic massage lotion or cream. Be sure to work the entire quadriceps area. Continue for about 5 minutes then switch places with your partner.

**Figure 13.4** Effleurage massage stroke on the quadriceps muscle.

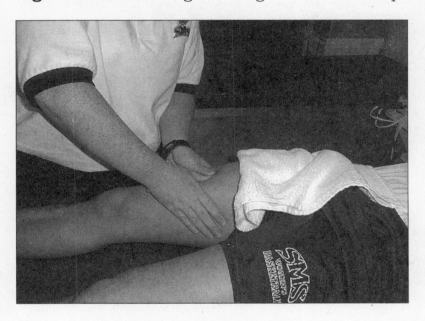

a) Once you have perfected the effleurage stroke, add pétrissage (kneading) and tapotement (hacking and slapping) strokes to your repertoire. Choose a different region of the body to perform these techniques, for example the calf, hamstrings, low back, or upper trapezius.

b) Friction massage is a technique that can be safely and effectively performed in an attempt to break up painful scar tissue/adhesions such as those that accompany tendinitis conditions. Position your lab partner supine on the treatment table with a towel roll under the knee joint to allow a slight bit of knee flexion. You should not have to use any massage lubricant (although you can if necessary). Perform a cross friction massage technique using your thumb only on the patellar tendon

(Figure 13.5). Perform this aggressively for 1 minute. You may also want to perform it on the biceps tendon running in the bicipital groove or over the IT band running laterally in the leg and attaching to Gerdy's tubercle. It is recommended that you only practice this technique for a total of 1 minute so as not to create too much uninjured tissue irritation in your partner.

**Figure 13.5** Cross-friction massage being applied to the patellar tendon.

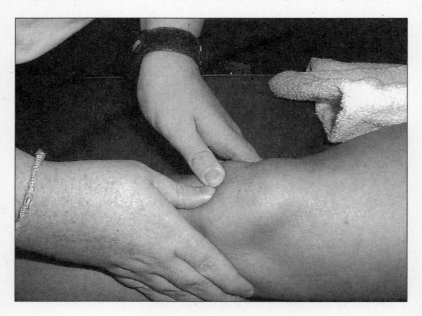

# *Laboratory Exercise 14*

# Aquatic Therapy
# in Rehabilitation

## PURPOSE:

The therapeutic effects of water have been well known for many years. Recently, more clinicians have realized the benefits of aquatic therapy and have incorporated water therapy routines into their rehabilitation plans. The purpose of this laboratory exercise is to review the foundational principles underlying aquatic therapy and to demonstrate various useful techniques that the student will then be able to incorporate into their own clinical programs.

## ATHLETIC TRAINING EDUCATIONAL COMPETENCIES:

*Therapeutic Exercise (Psychomotor Domain)*

- Demonstrates the appropriate application of contemporary therapeutic exercises including the following:

- Aquatic therapy

- Demonstrates the proper techniques for the performance of commonly prescribed rehabilitation and reconditioning exercises.

## ATHLETIC TRAINING CLINICAL PROFICIENCIES:

*Therapeutic Exercise (The student will demonstrate the ability to perform therapeutic exercises.)*

- Exercise to improve cardiorespiratory endurance.

- The student will demonstrate the ability to instruct the following activities:

  - Aquatic exercises for upper and lower body

## REVIEW OF PRINCIPLES:

The clinician who has access to a pool for aquatic therapy can add an extremely powerful rehabilitation tool to their clinical collection. Before designing and implementing an aquatic therapy program, the clinician must have an understanding of the properties of water and how they can best be utilized to benefit the injured athlete. In a water environment it is buoyancy and not gravity that is the guiding principle of movement. Buoyancy is the upward thrust that acts in the opposite direction of gravity.[1] The following list indicates the many therapeutic effects of buoyancy:[1]

- Assist, support, or resist a movement
- Increase ROM and flexibility
- Decreases joint stress (joint decompression)
- Increased support with less muscle guarding
- Improves functional ability

Another principle that needs consideration is that of specific gravity. Simply stated, objects with a specific gravity of < 1 will float, while those > 1 will sink. On average the human body has a specific gravity of between 0.95 – 0.97, thus enabling the body to float. Because the specific gravity is not uniform across the body, assistive-buoyancy devices are sometimes necessary to help the athlete/patient float.

The third and final concept that needs attention is that of resistive force. When a patient moves through the water, a variety of resistive forces are at work on the system. These include cohesive, bow, and drag forces (Figure 14.1).[2]

**Figure 14.1** Schematic drawing of bow and drag forces.

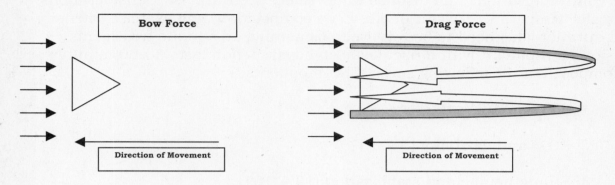

Cohesive forces run parallel to the water and are described as surface tension. The increase in water pressure where the front of the body interacts with the water best describes the bow force. Conversely, the drag force describes the decrease in water pressure at the rear of the body. Drag forces can be manipulated by changing the shape and speed of the object moving in the water.[2] The more streamlined the object, the lower the drag forces will be. Students are encouraged to do further exploration into the concepts of aquatic therapy by accessing the references listed at the end of this chapter.

Aquatic therapy has a number of physiological and psychological benefits. In most instances, rehabilitation exercises that can be performed on land can be introduced much sooner and can be more safe and effective in an aquatic environment. This is not only beneficial from a physical standpoint, but from a emotional one as well. The neuromuscular indications for aquatic interventions in a clinical setting include any of the following: [3]

- Decreased ROM
- Pain with movement/functional activity on land
- Balance, proprioception, and/or coordination deficits
- Decreased strength
- Weight-bearing restrictions on land
- Peripheral edema
- Gait deviations
- Poor movement patterns

Because a water-based rehabilitation plan poses greater risk to a patient, the clinician should consider a number of issues before initiating such an endeavor. Initially you should take a thorough patient history to determine any contraindications and discuss water safety precautions. Considerations for water temperature, water depth, body composition, and exercise intensity and duration also need to be reviewed. Generally, an aquatic treatment session for a patient with musculoskeletal dysfunction lasts 30-60 minutes and is composed of the following seven (7) components: [3]

1) Warm-up (5' – 15')

2) ROM and flexibility (5' – 15')

3) Strengthening and stabilization (13' – 15')

4) Endurance training (15' – 20')

5) Coordination, balance, and proprioception (5' – 15')

6) Functional activities (5' – 15')

7) Cool-down (5' – 15')

A clinician with a good imagination can develop a number of safe aquatic exercise routines to incorporate. A variety of commercially manufactured pool toys/devices can be used by the clinician to assist with their efforts. The following laboratory exercises will help the student to become proficient at using the aquatic environment for musculoskeletal rehabilitation purposes.

## TEXTBOOK REFERENCE CHAPTER:

Chapter 16

## REFERENCES:

1. Harvey, G. 1998. Why water? – Aquatic therapy makes a splash in sports medicine. *Sports Medicine Update* 13(2):14-23.

2. Hoogenboom, B., and N. Lomax. 2003. Aquatic therapy in rehabilitation. *Rehabilitation Techniques in Sports Medicine.* St. Louis: McGraw Hill.

3, Irion, J.M. Aquatic therapy. In *Therapeutic Exercise Techniques for Intervention* by Bandy, W.D., and B. Sanders. Baltimore, MD: Lippincott Williams & Wilkens.

# LABORATORY EXERCISES:

1. Let's begin by familiarizing ourselves with the tools of aquatic therapy. Look around the pool area or in the clinic to see what is available. A variety of devices can be utilized by the clinician to assist with buoyancy, resistance, stabilization, and positioning. The following is a list of tools that can be used in the aquatic environment:

- Kick boards
- Hand paddles
- Fins/flippers/water walkers
- Buoyancy cuffs
- Buoyancy vests/flotation devices (Aquajogger, WetVest, Aqua-sizer)
- Aqua gloves/webbed gloves
- Wonder boards
- Buoyancy dumbbells
- Milk jugs
- PVC pipe with soda bottles
- Flotation noodles
- Elastic tubing/rubber resistance bands
- Rubber medicine balls
- Head floats
- Underwater plastic board (AquaPlow)
- Resistance cuffs (various weights)
- Exercise bells

Try to become familiar with each device by gaining an understanding in regard to its purpose and function. Jump into the pool now and try it yourself!

2. Practical exposure and experience with the concepts underlying aquatic therapy will provide the student with a better understanding of the properties of water. This means that you'll have to get "wet"! Practice each of the following to further your understanding of the concepts of buoyancy and drag.

### a) Buoyancy

The ideal pool setting has water of different depths. The percent of the weight-bearing load will decrease with increased depth. In other words, the farther your body is submersed in water, the less the effect of gravity and the more the weight is "unloaded" from the body. You will see this as you float to the top of the water. Experiment by doing the following:

- Throw a tennis ball into the water. What happens? Why? (Remember specific gravity.)

- Throw a shot put into the water. What happens? Why?

- Stand upright and walk slowly from the shallow end (3') of the pool toward the deep end (6' to 8'), stopping every 4 to 5 feet. Do you begin to feel less of a load on your body the deeper you go? Once you get to a point where your neck is covered, turn around and go back to the shallow end. Do you now begin to experience the load returning to your body?

- Jump into the water wearing a life vest or other floatation device. What do you experience now? Do the same with two 5 lb ankle weights (cuffs) attached to your ankles. What happens now?

### b) Drag

- While standing in the shallow end, move the palm of one hand slowly through the water; turn your palm so that you're "chopping" at the water. Do you feel the drag? Experiment now by changing the palm face down and again move slowly though the water. Do you now experience more or less drag? Why?

- Now move your entire arm through the water as if performing the crawl stroke. Do you feel more or less drag? Perform the crawl stroke using an aqua glove or hand paddle. Does this increase or decrease drag? You should notice that the more streamlined an object is, the less drag, and vice versa.

3. There are a number of specific aquatic techniques that the student should become familiar with.  Each of these techniques can then be utilized in the rehabilitation of specific injuries or joint areas.  Keep in mind that the pool can also serve as a useful cardiovascular conditioning tool that can supplement any CV program.  Lap swimming and pool running with a flotation device are just two ways this can be accomplished.  Perform the following exercises in the pool:

a) Flexibility and Range of Motion

- Shoulder ROM (ABD, ADD, FLEX, EXT, IROT, EROT) exercises in the pool with and without a buoyancy cuff.  Stand shoulder-deep in the water.  Repeat on both arms.  You may also perform the Codman's shoulder exercise series in a similar format underwater.

- Knee ROM (FLEX, EXT) exercises in the pool with and without a buoyancy cuff.  Stand waist-deep in the water.  Repeat on both legs.

- Joint mobilization techniques can also be adopted for use in the water.  Try mobilizing the wrist (to improve flexion and extension) and ankle (to improve plantar and dorsiflexion) joints under water.

b) Gait Performance

- If the patient is unable to bear any weight, he can be placed supine in the water and, via active or active-assisted movements, he can perform walking patterns while floating.  Try this while wearing a flotation device or holding on to a flotation noodle.

- Vertical (upright) gait exercises can be performed by beginning in deep water and progressing to more shallow depths.  Pay close attention to executing proper gait patterns.

- Progression to stair walking in the water can be accomplished using either the pool steps or underwater benches/steps placed throughout the shallow  end in the pool.

- More advanced coordination activities can include braided sideways walking (underwater carioca), rocking horse exercise, stork standing positions, and underwater running

c) <u>Strengthening</u>

- Perform shoulder ROM while wearing a hand paddle or aqua glove. The motions can also be performed using elastic bands or tubing. Progression should include the incorporation of more functional movement patterns.

- Perform hip ROM exercises with resistance cuffs attached around the ankle or while wearing fins/flippers. The motions can also be performed using elastic bands or tubing. Progression should include the incorporation of more functional movement patterns. An example of this might be to have a soccer athlete perform the "scissors" kicking motion for 1 minute bouts with 30 seconds of rest between bouts.

- Quadriceps strengthening exercises might include:

- Mini-squats with the back to the wall
- Straight-leg kicks in the water
- Steps-ups on a ladder or step
- Walking backward while sitting on a kick board

d) <u>Functional Training</u>

Most functional activities can be simulated in a water environment. For example baseball throwing or tennis strokes can be accomplished underwater. Performing such activities in advance of land performance will increase proprioceptive awareness and build psychological confidence. Additionally, those involved in kicking or jumping sports will find a great many benefits to performing their skills underwater. Practice the following sporting maneuvers underwater:

- Tennis forehand stroke with a table tennis paddle
- Baseball throw while kneeling in the shallow water
- Soccer or football kick

# *Laboratory Exercise 15*

# Functional Progressions and Functional Testing in Rehabilitation

## PURPOSE:

Progression is defined as movement or advancement toward a specific goal. You may have heard the saying you must "crawl before you walk" or "walk before you can run"? The same holds true with functional progressions in rehabilitation. Typically these progressions culminate the rehabilitation journey as the athlete/patient makes his or her way to a return to activity or competition. The purpose of this laboratory exercise is to review the concept of functional progression and then develop ways in which you as the clinician can create and incorporate the progression components into a rehabilitation plan.

## ATHLETIC TRAINING EDUCATIONAL COMPETENCIES:

*Therapeutic Exercise (Psychomotor Domain)*

- Demonstrates the appropriate application of contemporary therapeutic exercises including the following:

  - Functional rehabilitation and reconditioning

- Demonstrates the proper techniques for the performance of commonly prescribed rehabilitation and reconditioning exercises.

- Performs a functional assessment for safe return to physical activity

# ATHLETIC TRAINING CLINICAL PROFICIENCIES:

*Therapeutic Exercise (The student will demonstrate the ability to perform therapeutic exercises.)*
>    - The student will demonstrate the ability to instruct and perform exercises to improve activity-specific skills (running, striking, throwing, catching, swimming, biking, climbing, etc...)

# REVIEW OF PRINCIPLES:

The term "functional" is an adjective that is defined as "having or performing a function." In the case of athletic rehabilitation, the word "functional" is used to describe activities that an athlete will need to perform in their specific sport endeavor. King defines function as referring to movement patterns that require motion from more than one joint and in more than one anatomical plane.[1] Traditionally, functional exercises have been incorporated into the rehabilitation program as the athlete/patient is nearing the end of the progression from acute injury status to return to play/activity status. Although used traditionally in this manner, some clinicians find it necessary to incorporate functional activities earlier in the rehabilitation sequence. This part of the rehabilitation process is especially challenging to the clinician but is equally rewarding. The process of functional progression can be thought of as first building a foundation which then leads to putting the final piece in at the top. From a rehabilitation standpoint that final piece becomes the safe and effective return to athletic activity and competition.

Functional rehabilitation techniques involve the use of multiple joints functioning as a whole in an attempt to refine neuromuscular coordination and performance. A functional progression is a succession of activities that simulate actual motor and sport skills. This enables the athlete to acquire or reacquire the skills needed to perform athletic endeavors safely and effectively.[2] Functional activities are meant to complement traditional rehabilitation activities, not replace them. The goals of functional progression include the restoration of: [2]

>    - Joint ROM
>    - Strength
>    - Proprioception
>    - Agility
>    - Confidence

In order to accomplish these goals, a series of activities that promote success and achievement while still challenging the athlete are incorporated. Decision for progression to the next phase should be based on individual results and performance rather than time factors (i.e. week five, day 10, etc...).[2]

It is important that the clinician have a thorough understanding of the demands of the specific sport the athlete is involved with. This will assist them as they develop functional activities into the rehabilitation program. Functional assessment will also aid the clinician in determining baseline status of the patient, which in turn can become the starting point for progression. Harter describes functional testing as an indirect measure of muscular strength and power.[3] Functional tests should be related to specific functional activities. Throughout this lab manual you have been introduced to and have practiced a variety of rehabilitation tools that can essentially be incorporated into a functional test battery. There are several methods for measuring functional performance of both the upper and lower extremities. The following is a list of some of the ways in which sport-specific function can be evaluated:

- Throwing velocity
- CKC Upper Extremity Stability Test (see Chapter 10)
- Joint position sense
- Kinesthesia
- Sprint time
- Agility tests
- Vertical jump
- Co-contraction tests
- Hopping tests
- Carioca test
- Shuttle runs
- Balance tests
- Subjective evaluations on functional performance

Additional information pertaining to functional progressions and functional exercise activities can be found in the references listed below. The primary objective of the following laboratory assignments is to introduce the student to upper and lower extremity functional exercises and to help them incorporate these exercises into a logical progression.

# TEXTBOOK REFERENCE CHAPTER:

Chapter 17

# REFERENCES:

1. King, M.A. 2000. Functional stability for the upper quarter. *Athletic Therapy Today* 5(2):17-21.

2. McGee, M. 2003. Functional progressions and functional testing in rehabilitation. *Rehabilitation Techniques in Sports Medicine.* St. Louis: McGraw Hill.

3. Harter, R. 1996. Clinical rationale for closed kinetic chain activities in functional testing and rehabilitation of ankle pathologies. *Journal of Sport Rehabilitation* 5(1):13-24.

4. Davies, G.J., and S. Dickoff-Hoffman. 1993. Neuromuscular testing and rehabilitation of the shoulder complex. *Journal of Orthopedic and Sports Physical Therapy* 18(2):449-458.

5. Wilk, K.E., W.T. Romaniello, S.M. Soscia, C.A. Arrigo, and J.R. Andrews. The relationship between subjective knee scores, isokinetic testing, and functional testing in the ACL-reconstructed knee. 1994. *Journal of Orthopedic and Sports Physical Therapy* 20(2):60-73.

6. Kirby, R.F. 1971. A simple test of agility. *Coach and Athlete* June:30-31.

7. Johnson, B.L., and J.L. Nelson. 1986. *Practical Measurements for Evaluation in Physical Education.* Minneapolis, MN: Burgess Publishing Company.

8. Lephart, S.M., D.H. Perrin, F.H.Fu, and K. Minger. 1991. Functional performance tests for the anterior cruciate ligament insufficient athlete. *Athletic Training, JNATA* 26(1):44-50.

## LABORATORY EXERCISES:

1. Functional testing provides the clinician with a picture of the athlete's capabilities to perform specific tasks related to sport performance. It will also give the clinician a starting point for progression through the rehabilitation plan. Working with your lab partner, perform the following functional tasks:

a) Assessment of Throwing Velocity (Upper Extremity)

You can assess this in one of two ways:

(1) Meet with the softball or baseball coach and try to secure a radar gun that will assess throwing velocity. Measure a total of five (5) throws from a standard pitching distance of 60' 6". The average of the 5 throws becomes the baseline value.

(2) If a radar gun is unavailable, a hand timing technique can be used. With this assessment you will record the time of the flight of the ball from release until it is caught. The process is the same as described in #1 above. Velocity can then be calculated by dividing the distance traveled by the time (v =d/t).

b) Functional Throwing Performance Index (Upper Extremity)

Davies and Dickoff-Hoffman used this test to assess functional performance (neuromuscular control) after injury.[4] The test is performed by having your partner toss a rubber playground ball into a 1' x 1' (0.30 m x 0.30 m) square target taped to the wall (Figure 15.1). Have them perform as many tosses as possible in 30 sec. Calculate a performance index by dividing the total number of throws by the number of throws that actually land inside the target (total throws ÷ strikes).

**Figure 15.1** Execution of the Functional Throwing Performance test.

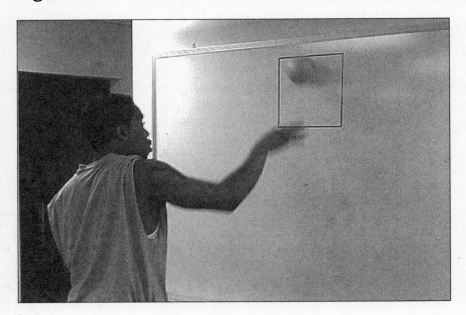

c) <u>Hopping Tests</u> (Lower Extremity)

Functional performance deficits of the lower extremity are commonly assessed using hop tests. The following three hop tests (Figure 15.2) are typically used:

**Figure 15.2** Functional hopping tests. (Reprinted from Wilk KE, Romaniello WT, Socia SM, Arrigo CA, Andrews JR. The relationship between subjective knee scores, isokinetic testing, and functional testing in the ACL-reconstructed knee. *J Ortho Sports Phys Ther.* 1994; 20(2):60-73, Figure 1, The three single-leg hop tests performed by the subjects, with permission of the Orthopaedic and Sports Sections of the American Physical Therapy Association.)

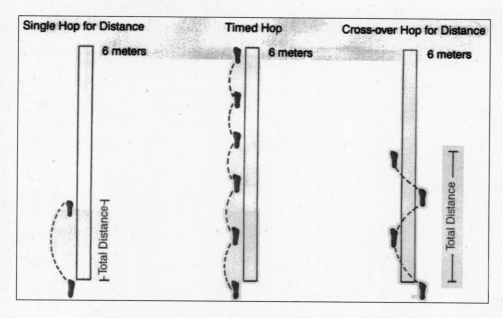

(1) *Single-Leg Hop for Distance* – Have your partner stand on one leg and hop as far forward as possible landing on the same leg. Measure the distance traveled. The average of three trials is used in calculating the limb symmetry score [5] (see description below). Perform the hops on both legs.

(2) *Single-Leg Timed Hop* – Instruct you lab partner to use explosive single-leg hops from start to finish across a distance of 6 meters. Record the time required to perform the task using the average of

three (3) trials to calculate the limb symmetry score. Perform the hops on both legs.

(3) _Single-Leg Cross-Over Triple Hop for Distance_ – Place a 15 cm wide strip of tape extending down the center of the 6 m hop course. This will designate the "center line." Have your partner hop three (3) consecutive times on the same foot crossing the center line with each hop. Measure the distance from the beginning to the third hop. The average of three trials is used to calculate the limb symmetry score. Perform the hops on both legs.

(4) _Limb Symmetry Score_ – To calculate the limb symmetry score, the mean score of the involved limb is divided by the mean time (or distance) of the uninvolved limb and the result multiplied by 100. A symmetry index of < 85% is usually considered abnormal.[5]

d) *SEMO Timed Agility Drill* (Lower Extremity)

The SEMO agility test incorporates forward, backward, and lateral running and is used to measure agility. This test was originally introduced by Kirby [6] and has been used extensively by physical educators for years. Performance is timed to the nearest .01 seconds. The test is conducted as shown in Figure 15.3 below. Complete the drill with a side shuffle from A to B, backpedal from B to D (diagonal cut), sprint from D to A, backpedal again from A to C, sprint from C to B, and side shuffle from B to A. Crossover steps are not allowed. The average time from three trials can be used as a baseline.

**Figure 15.3** Schematic representation of the SEMO agility drill. (reprinted with permission from Johnson & Nelson - Burgess Publishing Company, 1986 [7]).

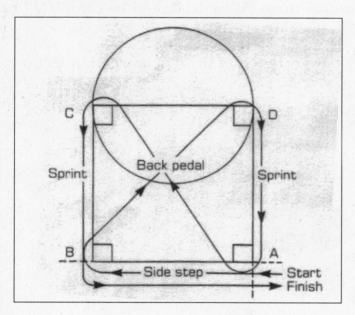

Normative values for women range from < 12.19 sec. to > 14.50 sec depending on fitness level. In males the times range from < 10.72 sec. to > 13.80 sec, again depending on fitness level.

e) *Co-contraction Test* (Lower Extremity)

This particular functional test was first described by Lephart et al. [8] as a test used to recreate the forces an athlete experiences during common sport skills/activities, and especially in those with ACL deficient knees. The test is set-up by securing a weight belt around the waist and attaching it to a 48" (122 cm) piece of heavy rubber tubing (1" diameter). The tubing is anchored 60" (152.5 cm) from the floor to a wall in front of the subject. A semi-circle with a radius of 96" (244 cm) from the wall anchor point is then placed on the floor using tape, paint, or chalk. The subject then stands facing the wall with toes touching the semi-circle line (this stretches the tubing beyond its' recoil length). The object of the test is to complete 5 wall-to-wall lengths (3 lengths right to left and 2 lengths left to right) as quickly as possible using a side shuffle pattern. (Do not use crossover steps.) Begin the test on the right side of the semi-circle (Figure 15.4). A total of three (3) trials should be completed with the average time used as a baseline.

**Figure 15.4** Schematic representation of the co-contraction test arc.

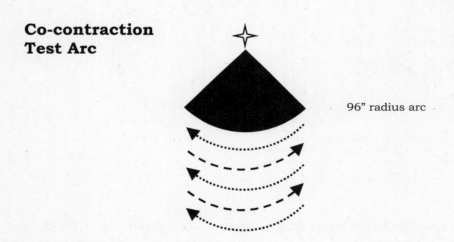

**Co-contraction Test Arc**

96" radius arc

2. The following are two case presentations: one for the upper extremity and another involving a lower extremity injury progression. For each case study you will be asked to develop a functional progression rehabilitation plan. The ultimate goal is a return to activity/competition for the injured athlete. For each case study you will be asked to:

- Make a list of a variety of functional tests that you might be able to use with the particular injury scenario.

- Describe what functional assessment tests you will need to complete in order for you as the clinician to get a baseline indication of the injured athlete's functional status.

- Outline your functional progression program based on sound logic and physiological/neuromuscular concepts. Keep in mind the interaction with the various phases of the inflammatory process. Additionally, it is important that you use the 5 goals of progression listed previously.

a) *Upper Extremity*

A 16 year-old male baseball player 12 weeks post-surgery for a rotator cuff repair of his left throwing shoulder: he has been involved in a clinical rehabilitation program for 6 weeks consisting of ROM exercises, inflammatory control, and minimal strengthening. He has been released by his physician to begin a functional progression toward complete recovery and an eventual return to throwing.

b) *Lower Extremity*

A 21 year-old female soccer player 4 weeks after a Grade 2-3 syndesmotic sprain of her right ankle: she has been immobilized in a walking cast for the last 4 weeks, and has tolerated weight-bearing quite nicely for the last 2 weeks. Her clinical rehabilitation program to date has consisted primarily of control of inflammation, limited ROM activity, controlled proprioception exercise, and a generalized cardiovascular conditioning routine. The team physician has requested that she begin a progression of functional activities in an attempt to return to playing once the playoffs begin.

# *Laboratory Exercise 16*

# Rehabilitation of Shoulder Injuries

## PURPOSE:

The purpose of this laboratory exercise is to enable the student an opportunity to incorporate each of the foundational concepts of rehabilitation (ROM, NM control, strength, flexibility, postural control, etc...) as they apply to specific shoulder injuries. The student will be asked to examine several case studies and to synthesize the rehabilitation techniques and principles they have learned into a concise and effective rehabilitation plan.

The following case scenarios are based on situations that an athletic trainer may encounter in various clinical settings, including a collegiate or high school athletic training room, a sports medicine clinic, and an industrial clinical setting. For each scenario, students should alternate taking on the role of athletic trainer with that of the injured athlete. The student in the role of the injured athlete should attempt to create an accurate simulation of the problem so that the partner (athletic trainer) can react accordingly. Most of the scenarios will involve creating proper documentation, including goal setting and exercise prescriptions.

## LABORATORY EXERCISES:

The following case studies relate to the rehabilitation of specific shoulder injuries. The student is asked to complete each of the tasks assigned to the scenario.

1. Ron is a 55 year-old competitive recreational tennis player who recently underwent a surgical repair of a SLAP lesion in his dominant left shoulder. He is now 8 days post-op and is seeing you to begin his rehabilitation. Your physical exam reveals three arthroscopy incisions that are healing well following the removal of sutures yesterday. His AROM is: 45° flexion, 10° extension, 30° abduction, 20° of external rotation, and 15° of internal rotation. All active motion is limited by pain. Manual muscle testing (MMT) reveals flexion *4-*, extension *5*, abduction *3+*, adduction *4*, external rotation *4-*, and internal rotation *3+* with all strength limitations due to pain. He is highly motivated to return to his tennis activities, which include playing in the state amateur tournament in four months.

A. Outline your rehabilitation program utilizing three distinct phases. Include at least three short term and three long term goals in each phase.

B. Write out two exercise prescriptions for PROM techniques to help restore range of motion during the initial phase of the rehabilitation program. Demonstrate your ability to instruct each of the exercise prescriptions and ensure they are performed correctly.

C. List three different techniques, including PNF, which could be utilized to restore strength levels during the third phase of the rehabilitation program. Write out two examples of exercise prescriptions for each technique. Demonstrate your ability to instruct each of the exercise prescriptions and ensure they are performed correctly.

D. With your lab partner, suggest slight modifications to each of the exercise prescriptions outlined in "B" above to make them more challenging to the athlete.

2. Eve is a 17 year-old high school volleyball player who has come to you complaining of persistent pain in her dominant right shoulder when she spikes the ball. The pain has been present for about three weeks and has been getting steadily worse during activity. She has also indicated a noticeable loss of motion. Physical exam reveals AROM limited by pain for all motions except extension, and her strength levels based on MMT show *4-* except for extension which is *5*. Your assessment of her other signs and symptoms leads you to suspect that she has an impingement syndrome.

A. List three different closed kinetic chain exercises you could utilize to restore normal strength levels. Write out a sample prescription for each exercise. Demonstrate your ability to instruct each of the exercise prescriptions and ensure they are performed correctly.

B. Assuming that she is continuing to participate, as tolerated list four short term goals you hope to accomplish over the next four weeks.

C. List three exercise prescriptions you could give to Eve for her to do in the swimming pool to maintain her cardiovascular fitness without aggravating her shoulder injury.

3. John is a 21 year-old college wrestler who sustained a GH joint dislocation to the right shoulder three weeks ago. Since this was his third dislocation in the past four years, he was immobilized by the team orthopedist for three weeks. He was cleared today by the team physician to begin rehabilitation with you. Your evaluation shows his PROM to be severely limited in all motions. He reports having no pain with active movements. His strength is rated at *4* in all planes of movement.

A. List four different techniques you could employ to restore range of motion, including joint mobilization and PNF. For each technique give two examples of exercise prescriptions. Demonstrate your ability to instruct each of the exercise prescriptions and ensure they are performed correctly.

B. List three different plyometric exercises you could incorporate during the final stage of rehabilitation. Write out three prescriptions for each exercise. Demonstrate your ability to instruct each of the exercise prescriptions and ensure they are performed correctly.

C.  With your lab partner, suggest slight modifications to each of the exercise prescriptions outlined in "B" above to make them more challenging to the athlete.

# *Laboratory Exercise 17*

# Rehabilitation of Elbow Injuries

## PURPOSE:

The purpose of this laboratory exercise is to enable the student an opportunity to incorporate each of the foundational concepts of rehabilitation (ROM, NM control, strength, flexibility, postural control, etc...) as they apply to specific elbow injuries. The student will be asked to examine several case studies and to synthesize the rehabilitation techniques and principles they have learned into a concise and effective rehabilitation plan.

The following case scenarios are based on situations that an athletic trainer may encounter in various clinical settings, including a collegiate or high school athletic training room, a sports medicine clinic, and an industrial clinical setting. For each scenario, students should alternate taking on the role of athletic trainer with that of the injured athlete. The student in the role of the injured athlete should attempt to create an accurate simulation of the problem so that the partner (athletic trainer) can react accordingly. Most of the scenarios will involve creating proper documentation, including goal setting and exercise prescriptions.

## LABORATORY EXERCISES:

The following case studies relate to the rehabilitation of specific elbow injuries. The student is asked to complete each of the tasks assigned to the scenario.

1. Ellen is a 44 year-old woman who attends an aerobic exercise class three times weekly. For the past week she has been experiencing pain over the lateral aspect of her left elbow. Over the course of the last two aerobics classes she has had difficulty gripping the dumbbells used in class. She denies any history of trauma but states that she helped her husband paint four rooms in their house two weeks ago. Your examination reveals pinpoint pain over the lateral epicondyle, pain with passive wrist flexion when the elbow is extended, and pain with resisted wrist extension.

A. Based on your examination, what do you think is wrong with Ellen? Describe the etiology of the condition.

B. Based on your answer above, list three long term goals for her rehabilitation.

C. List four different exercises you could utilize to address the problem. Write out prescriptions for each exercise. Demonstrate your ability to implement and/or instruct each of the four exercise prescriptions.

D. Write out five exercise prescriptions for Ellen to follow at home once she has completed her rehabilitation and returned to full activities. Demonstrate your ability to implement and /or instruct each of the five exercise prescriptions.

2. Mickey is a 22 year-old college baseball pitcher who over the summer underwent surgery to repair the ulnar collateral ligament of his pitching arm using the "Tommy John" procedure. He has been receiving therapy throughout the summer and is now returning to school. The treating physician has sent along a prescription for rehabilitation which simply reads "Evaluate and treat to increase strength and range of motion." Your initial evaluation reveals an extension lag of 10° yet you are able to achieve full passive extension. You suspect that Mickey's extension lag is due to inadequate accessory motions at the elbow.

A. List the accessory motions available at the elbow joint (humeroradial, humeroulnar, proximal radioulnar) and then list three different joint mobilization techniques you could perform to improve those accessory motions. Demonstrate the ability to correctly perform each exercise.

B. List four exercises designed to increase the muscular endurance of the extensor musculature and which would be appropriately used in the final stage of rehabilitation. Write out prescriptions for each exercise. Demonstrate your ability to implement and /or instruct each of the four exercise prescriptions.

C.  List three reactive training exercises designed to improve the proprioception in Mickey's throwing arm.  Write out prescriptions for each exercise. Demonstrate your ability to implement and /or instruct each of the three exercise prescriptions.

D.  Outline an interval throwing program to be used in the final stage of rehabilitation.

3. Ricki is a 20 year-old defensive tackle who sustained a dislocated elbow four weeks ago during the last football game of the season. He has been immobilized in a sling since the injury, but today the physician has allowed him to remove the sling and begin rehabilitation. Your evaluation shows total elbow range of motion to be from 40° to 100° of flexion, 5° each of pronation and supination, and *3+* strength in the elbow flexors and extensors.

A. Outline your rehabilitation program utilizing three distinct phases. Include at least two short term and two long term goals in each phase.

B. List three precautions to be aware of as the rehabilitation program is initiated and describe how these precautions will be addressed.

C. Write out four exercise prescriptions using both PROM and AROM techniques to help restore range of motion during the initial phase of the rehabilitation program. Demonstrate your ability to instruct each of the exercise prescriptions and ensure they are performed correctly.

D. Write out four exercise prescriptions using open and closed chain strengthening exercises which could be utilized during the second phase of the rehabilitation program. At least one exercise should incorporate the use of a Swiss ball. Demonstrate your ability to instruct each of the exercise prescriptions and ensure they are performed correctly.

# *Laboratory Exercise 18*

# Rehabilitation of Wrist, Hand, and Finger Injuries

## PURPOSE:

The purpose of this laboratory exercise is to enable the student an opportunity to incorporate each of the foundational concepts of rehabilitation (ROM, NM control, strength, flexibility, postural control, etc...) as they apply to specific wrist, hand, and finger injuries. The student will be asked to examine several case studies and to synthesize the rehabilitation techniques and principles they have learned into a concise and effective rehabilitation plan.

The following case scenarios are based on situations that an athletic trainer may encounter in various clinical settings, including a collegiate or high school athletic training room, a sports medicine clinic, or an industrial clinical setting. For each scenario, students should alternate taking on the role of athletic trainer with that of the injured athlete. The student in the role of the injured athlete should attempt to create an accurate simulation of the problem so that the partner (athletic trainer) can react accordingly. Most of the scenarios will involve creating proper documentation, including goal setting and exercise prescriptions.

## LABORATORY EXERCISES:

The following case studies relate to the rehabilitation of specific wrist, hand, and finger injuries. The student is asked to complete each of the tasks assigned to the scenario.

1. Tonya is a 23 year-old professional basketball player who underwent a surgical procedure involving a partial excision and debridement of the triangular fibrocartilage in the dominant right wrist eight days ago. She has been placed in a dynamic splint to facilitate flexion and referred to you for rehabilitation. Your evaluation reveals 10° extension, 15° of flexion, 5° of ulnar deviation, and 15° of radial deviation. Her strength levels are *3+* for wrist flexion, *3* for wrist extension and radial deviation, and *3-* for ulnar deviation.

A. Outline your rehabilitation program utilizing three distinct phases. Include at least two short term and two long term goals in each phase.

B. Describe three different aquatic therapy exercises which would be appropriate to increase range of motion during the initial phase of rehabilitation.

C.  List four strengthening exercise prescriptions that would be appropriate for the second stage of the rehabilitation program.  Demonstrate your ability to implement and /or instruct each of the exercise prescriptions.

D.  List four different functional tests based on objective criteria you could utilize to determine her readiness to return to unrestricted basketball activities.

2. Eric is a 33 year-old recreational bowler who underwent a surgical repair of a Boutonniere deformity of the PIP joint of the ring finger on his dominant hand four weeks ago. He has been in a splint which maintained the PIP joint in extension. The prescription from his physician asks you to begin gentle ROM and strengthening exercises for four weeks. You are also requested to devise a home exercise program. The splint is to be worn whenever Eric is not exercising.

A. List four exercise prescriptions designed to improve range of motion, including joint mobilizations. Demonstrate your ability to implement and /or instruct each of the exercise prescriptions.

B. List three exercise prescriptions which utilize rubber bands to strengthen the musculature of the fingers. Demonstrate your ability to implement and /or instruct each of the exercise prescriptions.

C. Create a home exercise program for Eric which includes at least three exercises to maintain/improve ROM and three exercises to increase strength. The exercises/activities should be different from the ones outlined above. Demonstrate your ability to implement and /or instruct each of the exercise prescriptions.

# *Laboratory Exercise 19*

# Rehabilitation of
# Groin, Hip, and Thigh Injuries

## **PURPOSE:**

The purpose of this laboratory exercise is to enable the student an opportunity
to incorporate each of the foundational concepts of rehabilitation (ROM, NM
control, strength, flexibility, postural control, etc...) as they apply to specific
groin, hip, and thigh injuries. The student will be asked to examine several
case studies and to synthesize the rehabilitation techniques and principles
they have learned into a concise and effective rehabilitation plan.

The following case scenarios are based on situations that an athletic trainer
may encounter in various clinical settings, including a collegiate or high school
athletic training room, a sports medicine clinic, or an industrial clinical setting.
For each scenario, students should alternate taking on the role of athletic
trainer with that of the injured athlete. The student in the role of the injured
athlete should attempt to create an accurate simulation of the problem so that
the partner (athletic trainer) can react accordingly. Most of the scenarios will
involve creating proper documentation, including goal setting and exercise
prescriptions.

176

## LABORATORY EXERCISES:

The following case studies relate to the rehabilitation of specific groin, hip, and thigh injuries. The student is asked to complete each of the tasks assigned to the scenario.

1. Jane is a 14 year-old high school track athlete who participates in the hurdles. Two days ago while practicing she felt a "pop" in the proximal aspect of her left hamstring. She currently has mild ecchymosis and pinpoint pain over the ischial tuberosity and into the proximal portion of the hamstring. She can perform a straight leg raise to 45° but is limited by pain. Her prone knee flexion strength is *3* and is also limited by pain. Your assessment is a Grade II hamstring strain.

A. Outline your rehabilitation program utilizing three distinct phases. Include at least two short term and two long term goals in each phase.

B. List two precautions to be aware of as the rehabilitation program is initiated and describe how these precautions will be addressed.

C. Write out four exercise prescriptions using PROM, AROM, and PNF techniques to help restore range of motion during the initial phase of the rehabilitation program. Demonstrate your ability to instruct each of the exercise prescriptions and ensure they are performed correctly.

D. Write out four exercise prescriptions using isometric and isotonic exercises to restore normal strength levels during the final stage of the rehabilitation program. Demonstrate your ability to instruct each of the exercise prescriptions and ensure they are performed correctly.

2. Robert is a 40 year-old recreational basketball player who sustained a contusion to his right anterior thigh two weeks ago. He indicates that he has been icing his thigh daily and walking with crutches most of the time. On examination today, he has a palpable mass in the mid-anterior thigh but no ecchymosis. His active range of motion and strength at the hip and knee are limited primarily due to pain.

A. Write out four exercise prescriptions using both PROM and AROM techniques to help restore range of motion during the initial phase of the rehabilitation program. Demonstrate your ability to instruct each of the exercise prescriptions and ensure they are performed correctly.

B. Write out two exercise prescriptions using muscle energy techniques to help restore range of motion at the hip and knee during the final stage of the rehabilitation program. Demonstrate your ability to instruct each of the exercise prescriptions and ensure they are performed correctly.

C.  Write out three exercise prescriptions for exercises/activities to improve Robert's cardiovascular endurance throughout the latter stages of his rehabilitation.  Demonstrate your ability to instruct each of the exercise prescriptions and ensure they are performed correctly.

3. Janet is a 12 year-old competitive AAU basketball player who has come to see you about a recurrent "popping" sensation in her right hip. Your assessment leads you to believe she has "snapping hip syndrome". You explain to her that it is not a serious condition and occurs primarily in young, rapidly growing adolescents. You decide to give her a home exercise program.

A. Write out a home exercise program containing only five exercises which will address her condition. Demonstrate your ability to instruct each of the exercise prescriptions and ensure they are performed correctly.

B. With your lab partner, suggest slight modifications to each of the exercise prescriptions outlined above to make them more challenging to the athlete.

4. John is a golfer who complains of intermittent pain in his left buttock and posterior leg. It has been bothering him for several weeks. He denies any history of trauma. Your assessment leads you to believe that he is suffering from piriformis syndrome.

A. Outline your approach to John's problem. Indicate what you feel needs to be addressed in his rehabilitation program and how you plan on addressing those needs. Include at least four appropriate exercise interventions and prescriptions for those interventions. Demonstrate your ability to instruct each of the exercise prescriptions and ensure they are performed correctly.

# *Laboratory Exercise 20*

# Rehabilitation of
# Knee Injuries

## PURPOSE:

The purpose of this laboratory exercise is to enable the student an opportunity to incorporate each of the foundational concepts of rehabilitation (ROM, NM control, strength, flexibility, postural control, etc...) as they apply to specific knee injuries. The student will be asked to examine several case studies and to synthesize the rehabilitation techniques and principles they have learned into a concise and effective rehabilitation plan.

The following case scenarios are based on situations that an athletic trainer may encounter in various clinical settings, including a collegiate or high school athletic training room, a sports medicine clinic, or an industrial clinical setting. For each scenario, students should alternate taking on the role of athletic trainer with that of the injured athlete. The student in the role of the injured athlete should attempt to create an accurate simulation of the problem so that the partner (athletic trainer) can react accordingly. Most of the scenarios will involve creating proper documentation, including goal setting and exercise prescriptions.

## LABORATORY EXERCISES:

The following case studies relate to the rehabilitation of specific knee injuries. The student is asked to complete each of the tasks assigned to the scenario.

1. Jason is a 20 year-old wide receiver who underwent a reconstruction procedure for an anterior cruciate ligament tear in his left knee two days ago. His surgery involved utilizing a patellar tendon graft from the left leg. He is currently PWB with crutches. The team orthopedist has told you to begin rehabilitation today. You plan to see Jason daily in the training room.

A. List five activities or exercises that you will have Jason perform over the next three weeks. Write three objective goals for this early stage of the rehabilitation program. Demonstrate your ability to instruct each of the activities or exercise prescriptions and ensure they are performed correctly.

B. Eight weeks have passed and Jason is now FWB without a limp, has full extension, and flexes the knee to 120°. Write three objective goals for this stage of the rehabilitation program. Addressing these goals, list five activities or exercises, including balance and proprioceptive activities, that you will have Jason perform over the next two months. Demonstrate your ability to instruct each of the activities or exercise prescriptions and ensure they are performed correctly.

C. At six months post-op you and the team orthopedist feel that Jason may be ready to be released to full activity. List five different functional tests based on objective criteria you could utilize to determine his readiness to return to unrestricted football activities.

D. The team orthopedist would also like to have an isokinetic test performed on Jason prior to releasing him. List five performance criteria you would look for in the results of the isokinetic test and indicate any available normative data to be used for comparisons.

2. Erin is a 18 year-old freshman cross country runner who is complaining of right lateral knee pain which has been getting worse over the last three weeks. Your evaluation of her knee leads you to conclude that she has iliotibial band friction syndrome. You decide to hold her out from practice for 7-10 days and monitor her rehabilitation in the training room.

A. List three objective goals for your rehabilitation program during the next two weeks.

B. List three different exercise prescriptions which will address her flexibility and muscular endurance over the next two weeks. Demonstrate your ability to instruct each of the exercise prescriptions and ensure they are performed correctly.

C.  List two different activities or exercises you will have Erin perform in order to maintain her cardiovascular fitness while she is not running.  Demonstrate your ability to instruct each of the activities or exercise and ensure they are performed correctly.

3. Karen is a 14 year-old junior high school basketball player who is complaining of anterior knee pain that has gotten progressively worse since basketball practice started two weeks ago. Your evaluation reveals full knee motion, retropatellar pain with resisted terminal knee extension, mild crepitus, atrophy of the vastus medialis, and tight hamstrings and calves. You conclude that Karen is suffering from patellofemoral compression syndrome.

A. Outline your rehabilitation program and include at least four goals for the next four weeks.

B. List three exercise prescriptions, including at least one that utilizes muscle energy techniques, to address her decreased flexibility. Demonstrate your ability to instruct each of the exercise prescriptions and ensure they are performed correctly.

C.  List three exercise prescriptions to address her decreased quad strength. Demonstrate your ability to instruct each of the exercise prescriptions and ensure they are performed correctly.

D.  Write out a home exercise program which will address her condition. Demonstrate your ability to instruct each of the exercise prescriptions and ensure they are performed correctly.

# *Laboratory Exercise 21*

# Rehabilitation of Lower-Leg Injuries

## PURPOSE:

The purpose of this laboratory exercise is to enable the student an opportunity to incorporate each of the foundational concepts of rehabilitation (ROM, NM control, strength, flexibility, postural control, etc...) as they apply to specific lower-leg injuries. The student will be asked to examine several case studies and to synthesize the rehabilitation techniques and principles they have learned into a concise and effective rehabilitation plan.

The following case scenarios are based on situations that an athletic trainer may encounter in various clinical settings, including a collegiate or high school athletic training room, a sports medicine clinic, or an industrial clinical setting. For each scenario, students should alternate taking on the role of athletic trainer with that of the injured athlete. The student in the role of the injured athlete should attempt to create an accurate simulation of the problem so that the partner (athletic trainer) can react accordingly. Most of the scenarios will involve creating proper documentation, including goal setting and exercise prescriptions.

## LABORATORY EXERCISES:

The following case studies relate to the rehabilitation of specific lower-leg injuries. The student is asked to complete each of the tasks assigned to the scenario.

1. Adam is a 16 year-old young man who recently began training for a charity marathon to be held four months from now. He has had no prior experience with running. He states that after running about 2 miles every other day for two weeks he has developed pain along the medial distal tibia. The pain previously occurred about 15 minutes into his run but he has noted that recently it is beginning to hurt within the first 3-4 minutes and persists throughout his run. Your evaluation finds pain with palpation along the distal third of the medial tibia, a grade of 4 with MMT of the anterior and posterior tibialis muscles, and 5 degrees of active dorsiflexion. Your assessment is medial tibial stress syndrome, also known as "shin splints."

A. Outline your rehabilitation program and include at least four goals for the next four weeks.

B. Write two exercise prescriptions which address each of the four goals. Demonstrate your ability to instruct each of the exercise prescriptions and ensure they are performed correctly.

C. Write out a sample training schedule for Adam to follow after you release him to resume running.

2. Denise is a 45 year-old recreational tennis player who suffered a ruptured left Achilles tendon while playing and underwent a surgical repair three weeks ago. Since she is on the faculty at your university, you have agreed to perform her rehabilitation. Her physician has sent along a note stating that he would like you to begin range of motion activities, progress her to strengthening exercises, and gradually return her to tennis activities. She has been immobilized in 10° of plantar flexion until today. She is PWB with her crutches. You note considerable muscle atrophy in the left lower leg. She has 50° of plantar flexion and 20° of inversion and eversion.

A. Outline your rehabilitation program utilizing three distinct phases. Include at least two short term and two long term goals in each phase.

B. Write out four exercise prescriptions using both PROM and AROM techniques to help restore range of motion during the initial phase of the rehabilitation program. Demonstrate your ability to instruct each of the exercise prescriptions and ensure they are performed correctly.

C.  Write out an exercise prescription for joint mobilization to increase dorsiflexion.  Demonstrate the ability to correctly administer the joint mobilization prescription.

D.  Write out an exercise prescription for three exercises Denise can do in the swimming pool on her own.  Demonstrate your ability to instruct each of the exercise prescriptions.

# *Laboratory Exercise 22*

# Rehabilitation of
# Ankle and Foot Injuries

## PURPOSE:

The purpose of this laboratory exercise is to enable the student an opportunity to incorporate each of the foundational concepts of rehabilitation (ROM, NM control, strength, flexibility, postural control, etc...) as they apply to specific ankle and foot injuries. The student will be asked to examine several case studies and to synthesize the rehabilitation techniques and principles they have learned into a concise and effective rehabilitation plan.

The following case scenarios are based on situations that an athletic trainer may encounter in various clinical settings, including a collegiate or high school athletic training room, a sports medicine clinic, or an industrial clinical setting. For each scenario, students should alternate taking on the role of athletic trainer with that of the injured athlete. The student in the role of the injured athlete should attempt to create an accurate simulation of the problem so that the partner (athletic trainer) can react accordingly. Most of the scenarios will involve creating proper documentation, including goal setting and exercise prescriptions.

## LABORATORY EXERCISES:

The following case studies relate to the rehabilitation of specific ankle and foot injuries. The student is asked to complete each of the tasks assigned to the scenario.

1. Jeff is a 18 year-old high school senior who suffered a second degree lateral ankle sprain yesterday while participating in pre-season basketball drills. He has a history of four previous sprains but none were this severe. X-rays taken to rule out fracture were negative. Practice begins in six weeks and he is very anxious to be ready at that time.

A. Outline your rehabilitation program utilizing three distinct phases. Include at least two short term and two long term goals in each phase.

B. List three reactive training exercises designed to improve the proprioception in Jeff's ankle. Write out prescriptions for each exercise. Demonstrate your ability to implement and /or instruct each of the three exercise prescriptions.

C.  With your lab partner, suggest modifications to each of the exercise prescriptions outlined above to make them more challenging to the athlete.

D.  List four different functional tests based on objective criteria you could utilize to determine his readiness to return to basketball activities with no restrictions.

2. Leslie is an administrative secretary who has developed recurrent plantar fasciitis in the left foot. She notes that her symptoms increase if she wears certain shoes or has to climb stairs on several occasions during the work day. Your evaluation indicates a pes cavus foot, pinpoint pain with palpation over the insertion of the plantar fascia at the medial tubercle of the calcaneus, and 5° of dorsiflexion.

A. Outline a home care program for plantar fasciitis which includes five activities or exercises. Indicate your rationale for each activity or exercise and how you feel each will improve her condition.

B. List three other interventions you could recommend for Leslie. Provide appropriate rationale for each recommendation.

# *Laboratory Exercise 23*

# Rehabilitation of Injuries to the Spine

## PURPOSE:

The purpose of this laboratory exercise is to enable the student an opportunity to incorporate each of the foundational concepts of rehabilitation (ROM, NM control, strength, flexibility, postural control, etc...) as they apply to specific injuries to the spine. The student will be asked to examine several case studies and to synthesize the rehabilitation techniques and principles they have learned into a concise and effective rehabilitation plan.

The following case scenarios are based on situations that an athletic trainer may encounter in various clinical settings, including a collegiate or high school athletic training room, a sports medicine clinic, or an industrial clinical setting. For each scenario, students should alternate taking on the role of athletic trainer with that of the injured athlete. The student in the role of the injured athlete should attempt to create an accurate simulation of the problem so that the partner (athletic trainer) can react accordingly. Most of the scenarios will involve creating proper documentation, including goal setting and exercise prescriptions.

## LABORATORY EXERCISES:

The following case studies relate to the rehabilitation of specific injuries to the spine. The student is asked to complete each of the tasks assigned to the scenario.

1. Formulate a core stabilization program for Justin, a 20 year-old college basketball player who recently transferred to your school and has a long history of intermittent low back pain. There is no known neurological involvement and a normal radiological history.

A. Write out four prescriptions for exercises that can be performed on the treatment table (plinth). Demonstrate your ability to instruct each of the exercise prescriptions and ensure they are performed correctly.

B. Write out four prescriptions for exercises to be done with a Swiss ball. Demonstrate your ability to instruct each of the exercise prescriptions and ensure they are performed correctly.

C.  Write our four prescriptions for exercises to be done with foam rolls of various sizes.  Demonstrate your ability to instruct each of the exercise prescriptions and ensure they are performed correctly.

D.  Formulate a strength and flexibility program for Justin using four different PNF techniques.  Write out appropriate exercise prescriptions for each PNF technique.  Demonstrate the ability to correctly administer each prescription.

E. Formulate an aquatic therapy program for Justin which will address core stability and endurance activities.  Write out five appropriate exercise prescriptions and provide rationale for each prescription.

# NOTES

# NOTES

# NOTES

# NOTES

# NOTES

# NOTES

# NOTES

# NOTES

# NOTES

# NOTES

# NOTES

# NOTES